PLANS OF CARE FOR
SPECIALTY PRACTICE

Cardiovascular Critical Care Nursing

PLANS OF CARE FOR
SPECIALTY PRACTICE

Cardiovascular Critical Care Nursing

DIANE K. DRESSLER, RN, MSN, CCRN, CCTC
Senior Clinical Transplant Coordinator
St. Luke's Medical Center
Milwaukee, Wisconsin

KATHY V. GETTRUST, RN, BSN ~ *Series Editor*
Case Manager
Midwest Medical Home Care
Milwaukee, Wisconsin

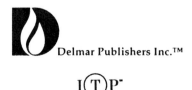

Delmar Publishers Inc.™

I(T)P⁻

NOTICE TO THE READER

Publisher does not warrant or guarantee any of the products described herein or perform any independent analysis in connection with any of the product information contained herein. Publisher does not assume, and expressly disclaims, any obligation to obtain and include information other than that provided to it by the manufacturer.

The reader is expressly warned to consider and adopt all safety precautions that might be indicated by the activities described herein and to avoid all potential hazards. By following the instructions contained herein, the reader willingly assumes all risks in connection with such instructions.

The publisher makes no representations or warranties of any kind, including but not limited to, the warranties of fitness for particular purpose or merchantability, nor are any such representations implied with respect to the material set forth herein, and the publisher takes no responsibility with respect to such material. The publisher shall not be liable for any special, consequential or exemplary damages resulting, in whole or in part, from the readers' use of, or reliance upon, this material.

Delmar publishing team:
Publisher: David C. Gordon
Administrative Editor: Patricia Casey
Associate Editor: Elisabeth F. Williams
Project Editor: Danya M. Plotsky
Production Coordinator: Mary Ellen Black
Art and Design Coordinator: Megan K. DeSantis
                            Timothy J. Conners

For information, address

Delmar Publishers Inc.
3 Columbia Circle, Box 15015,
Albany, NY 12212-5015

Printed in the United States of America
Published simultaneously in Canada
by Nelson Canada,
a division of The Thomson Corporation

1 2 3 4 5 6 7 8 9 10 XXX 00 99 98 97 96 95 94

Library of Congress Cataloging-in-Publication Data

Dressler, Diane K.
    Cardiovascular critical care nursing / Diane K. Dressler.
       p. cm.—(Plans of care for specialty practice)
    Includes index.
    ISBN 0-8273-5712-5
    1. Cardiovascular system—Diseases—Nursing. 2. Intensive care nursing. I. Title. II. Series.
       [DNLM: 1. Cardiovascular Diseases—nursing. 2. Critical Care—nurses' instruction.   WY 152.5 D773c 1994]
    RC674.D74   1994
    610.73'691—dc20
    DNLM/DLC
    for Library of Congress   93-22631
                                                                                    CIP

TABLE OF CONTENTS

CONTRIBUTORS

Patricia A. Burke, RN, MS, CCRN
Clinical Nurse Specialist
Midwest Heart Surgery Institute, Ltd.
Milwaukee, Wisconsin
- Angina Pectoris
- Cardiac Tamponade
- Hypertensive Crisis

Diane K. Dressler, RN, MSN, CCRN,
  CCTC
Senior Clinical Transplant Coordinator
St. Luke's Medical Center
Milwaukee, Wisconsin
- Cardiac Transplantation

Claire C. Elsesser, RN, BSN, CCRN
Nurse Clinician, Cardiovascular
  Surgical Intensive Care Unit
St. Luke's Medical Center
Milwaukee, Wisconsin
- Cardiac Surgery: Acute Perioperative
  Period
- Ventricular Assist Device

Maurice H. Espinoza, RN, MSN
Staff Nurse, Cardiovascular Surgical
  Intensive Care Unit
St. Luke's Medical Center
Milwaukee, Wisconsin
- Cardiomyopathy and Myocarditis

Rita E. Herman, RN, MSN
Clinical Nurse Specialist, Mental Health
  Services
St. Luke's Medical Center
Milwaukee, Wisconsin
- Coping with Cardiac Crises

Lori A. Hislop, RN, BSN, CCRN
Staff Nurse, Thoracic Transplant
  Unit
St. Luke's Medical Center
Milwaukee, Wisconsin
- Percutaneous Transluminal
  Coronary Angioplasty
- Peripheral Vascular Disease

Dona L. Hutson, RN, BSN
Staff Nurse, Cardiovascular Surgical
  Intermediate Care Unit
St. Luke's Medical Center
Milwaukee, Wisconsin
- Cardiac Surgery: Recovery Period

Sandra A. Kopczenski, RN, BSN
Critical Care Nurse Clinician
St. Luke's Medical Center
Milwaukee, Wisconsin
- Cerebral Vascular Accident

Alice T. Kramer, RN, BSN, MS,
  CEN
Clinical Nurse Specialist, Emergency
  Services
St. Luke's Medical Center
Milwaukee, Wisconsin
- Thrombolytic Therapy

Linda M. Lundin, RN
Cardiac Nurse Clinician
St. Luke's Medical Center
Milwaukee, Wisconsin
- Artificial Cardiac Pacing

Mary G. Schigoda, RN, MSN, CCRN
Clinical Nurse Specialist
Thoracic Transplant Unit
St. Luke's Medical Center
Milwaukee, Wisconsin
- Acute Myocardial Infarction
- Cardiogenic Shock
- Congestive Heart Failure

Cherri A. Schleicher, RN, BSN, CCRN
Nurse Clinician
Arrhythmia Consultants of Milwaukee
Milwaukee, Wisconsin
- Implantable Cardioverter Defibrillator

Julie A. Sommer, RN, MSN
Clinical Transplant Coordinator
St. Luke's Medical Center
Milwaukee, Wisconsin
- Aortic Aneurysm Repair
- Infective Endocarditis: Acute/Subacute

Sandra L. Zemke, RN, BSN
Staff Nurse, Cardiac Rehabilitation
St. Luke's Medical Center
Milwaukee, Wisconsin
- Cardiac Rehabilitation

PREFACE

In the specialty practice area of cardiovascular critical care, there are continuous advancements in the diagnostic procedures and treatment modalities for cardiovascular conditions. In conjunction with new techniques such as electrophysiology testing and implantable cardioverter defibrillators, the nursing care of these patients has become increasingly complex, requiring a high level of technical knowledge and skill.

Cardiovascular Critical Care is a reference text containing nursing care plans pertinent to the conditions and disorders seen most commonly in this specialty setting. The care plans address both clinical conditions (such as acute myocardial infarction) and therapeutic interventions (such as artificial cardiac pacing). The plans can be used to assist practicing critical care nurses to organize and implement the care of patients with complex cardiovascular problems. Using current NANDA nursing diagnoses whenever possible, the chapters succinctly but completely describe each clinical problem and the nursing diagnoses most commonly associated with it. Specific nursing interventions are outlined to direct the assessment, implementation, and evaluation of nursing care. In addition, rationales for specific interventions are included to emphasize the scientific basis for nursing intervention.

The care plans were written by fourteen practicing specialists in cardiovascular critical care, who are associated with the cardiovascular services of St. Luke's Medical Center in Milwaukee, Wisconsin. Authors were chosen for their clinical expertise, experience, and effectiveness in managing complex cardiovascular problems. The care plans will be helpful to critical care nurses in many settings from the emergency room to home health care. They may be especially helpful to nurses who do not have recent experience with a particular clinical problem or therapeutic intervention. It is recognized that there may be regional differences in patient care management protocols, and an attempt was made to be as universal as possible.

It is with pleasure that we welcome you to utilize our care plans as you approach the patient with a complex cardiovascular problem. We sincerely hope that you will enjoy using the plans and that they will be of benefit to you and your patients.

SERIES INTRODUCTION

Scientific and technological developments over the past several decades have revolutionized health care and care of the sick. These rapid and extensive advancements of knowledge have occurred in all fields, necessitating an ever-increasing specialization of practice. For nurses to be effective and meet the challenge in today's specialty settings, the body of clinical knowledge and skill needs to continually expand. *Plans of Care for Specialty Practice* has been written to aid the practicing nurse in meeting this challenge. The purpose of this series is to provide comprehensive, state-of-the-art plans of care and associated resource information for patient situations most commonly seen within a specialty that will serve as a standard from which care can be individualized. These plans of care are based on the profession's scientific approach to problem solving—the nursing process. Though the books are primarily written as a guide for frontline staff nurses and clinical nurse specialists practicing in specialty settings, they have application for student nurses as well.

DOCUMENTATION OF CARE

The Joint Commission on Accreditation of Healthcare Organizations (JCAHO) assumes authority for evaluating the quality and effectiveness of the practice of nursing. In 1991, the JCAHO developed its first new nursing care standards in more than a decade. One of the changes brought about by these new standards was the elimination of need for every patient to have a handwritten or computer-generated care plan in his or her chart detailing all or most of the care to be provided. The Joint Commission's standard that describes the documentation requirements stipulates that nursing assessments, identification of nursing diagnoses and/or patient care needs, interventions, outcomes of care, and discharge planning be permanently integrated into the clinical record. In other words, the nursing process needs to be documented. A separate care plan is no longer needed; however, planning and implementing care must continue as always, but using whatever form of documentation that has been approved by an institution. *Plans of Care for Specialty Practice* can be easily used with a wide variety of approaches to documentation of care.

ELEMENTS OF THE PLANS OF CARE

The chapter title is the presenting situation, which represents the most commonly seen conditions/disorders treated within the specialty setting. It may be a medical diagnosis (e.g., diabetes mellitus), a syndrome (e.g., acquired immunodeficiency syndrome), a surgical procedure (e.g., mastectomy), or a diagnostic/therapeutic procedure (e.g., thrombolytic therapy).

An opening paragraph provides a definition or concise overview of the presenting situation. It describes the condition and may contain pertinent physiological/psychological bases for the disorder. It is brief and not intended to replace further investigation for comprehensive understanding of the condition.

Etiologies

A listing of causative factors responsible for or contributing to the presenting situation is provided. This may include predisposing diseases, injuries or trauma, surgeries, microorganisms, genetic factors, environmental hazards, drugs, or psychosocial disorders. In presenting situations where no clear causal relationship can be established, current theories regarding the etiology may be included.

Clinical Manifestations

Objective and subjective signs and symptoms which describe the particular presenting situation are included. This information is revealed as a result of a health history and physical assessment and becomes part of the data base.

Clinical/Diagnostic Findings

This component contains possible diagnostic tests and procedures which might be done to determine abnormalities associated with a particular presenting situation. The name of the diagnostic procedure and the usual abnormal findings are listed.

Nursing Diagnosis

The nursing management of the health problem commences with the planning care phase of the nursing process. This includes obtaining a comprehensive history and physical assessment, identification of the nursing diagnoses, expected outcomes, interventions, and discharge planning needs.

Diagnostic labels identified by NANDA through the Tenth National Conference in April 1992 are being used throughout this series. (Based on North American Nursing Diagnosis Association, 1992. *NANDA Nursing Diagnoses: Definitions and Classification 1992.*) We have also identified new diagnoses not yet on the official NANDA list. We endorse NANDA's recommendation for nurses to develop new nursing diagnoses as the need arises and we encourage nurses using this series to do the same.

"Related to" Statements

Related to statements suggest a link or connection to the nursing diagnosis and provide direction for identifying appropriate nursing interventions. They are termed contributing factors, causes, or etiologies. There is frequently more than one related to statement for a given diagnosis. For example, change in job, marital difficulties, and impending surgery may all be "related to" the patient's nursing diagnosis of anxiety.

There is disagreement at present regarding inclusion of pathophysiological/medical diagnoses in the list of related to statements. Frequently, a medical diagnosis does not provide adequate direction for nursing care. For example, the nursing diagnosis of chronic pain related to rheumatoid arthritis does not readily suggest specific nursing interventions. It is more useful for the nurse to identify specific causes of the chronic pain such as inflammation, swelling, and fatigue; these in turn suggest more specific interventions. In cases where the medical diagnosis provides the best available information, as occurs with the more medically oriented diagnoses such as decreased cardiac output or impaired gas exchange, the medical terminology is included.

Defining Characteristics

Data collection is frequently the source for identifying defining characteristics, sometimes called signs and symptoms or patient behaviors. These data, both subjective and objective, are organized into meaningful patterns and used to verify the nursing diagnosis. The most commonly seen defining characteristics for a given diagnosis are included and should not be viewed as an all-inclusive listing.

Risk Factors

Nursing diagnoses designated as high risk are supported by risk factors that direct nursing actions to reduce or prevent the problem from developing. Since these nursing diagnoses have not yet occurred, risk factors replace the listing of actual defining characteristics and related to statements.

Patient Outcomes

Patient outcomes, sometimes termed patient goals, are observable behaviors or data which measure changes in the condition of the patient after nursing treatment. They are objective indicators of progress toward prevention of the development of high-risk nursing diagnoses or resolution/modification of actual diagnoses. Like other elements of the plan of care, patient outcome statements are dynamic and must be reviewed and modified periodically as the patient progresses. Assigning realistic "target or evaluation dates" for evaluation of progress toward outcome achievement is crucial. Since there are so many considerations involved in when the outcome could be achieved (e.g., varying lengths of stay, individual patient condition), these plans of care do not include evaluation dates; the date needs to be individualized and assigned using the professional judgment and discretion of the nurse caring for the patient.

Nursing Interventions

Nursing interventions are the treatment options/actions the nurse employs to prevent, modify, or resolve the nursing diagnosis. They are driven by the related to statements and risk factors and are selected based on the outcomes to be achieved. Treatment options should be chosen only if they apply realistically to a specific patient condition. The nurse also needs to determine frequencies for each intervention based on professional judgment and individual patient need.

We have included independent, interdependent, and dependent nursing interventions as they reflect current practice. We have not made a distinction between these kinds of interventions because of institutional differences and increasing independence in nursing practice. The interventions that are interdependent or dependent will require collaboration with other professionals. The nurse will need to determine when this is necessary and take appropriate action. The interventions include assessment, therapeutic, and teaching actions.

Rationales

The rationales provide scientific explanation or theoretical bases for the interventions; interventions can then be selected more intelligently and actions can be tailored to each individual's needs.

The rationales provided may be used as a quick reference for the nurse unfamiliar with the reason for a given intervention and as a tool for patient education. These rationales may include principles, theory, and/or research findings from current literature. The rationales are intended as reference information and, as such, should not be transcribed into the permanent patient record. A rationale is not provided when the intervention is self-explanatory.

Discharge Planning/Continuity of Care

Because stays in acute care hospitals are becoming shorter due to cost containment efforts, patients are frequently discharged still needing care; discharge planning is the process of anticipating and planning for needs after discharge. Effective discharge planning begins with admission and continues with ongoing assessment of the patient and family needs. Included in the discharge planning/continuity of care section are suggestions for follow-up measures, such as skilled nursing care; physical, occupational, speech, or psychiatric therapy; spiritual counseling, social service assistence; follow-up appointments, and equipment/supplies.

References

A listing of references appears at the conclusion of each plan of care or related group of plans. The purpose of the references is to cite specific work used and to specify background information or suggestions for further reading. Citings provided represent the most current nursing theory and/or research bases for inclusion in the plans of care.

A Word About Family

The authors and editors of this series recognize the vital role that family and/or other significant people play in the recovery of a patient. Isolation from the family unit during hospitalization may disrupt self-concept and feelings of security. Family members, or persons involved in the patient's care, must be included in the teaching to ensure that it is appropriate and will be followed. In an effort to constrain the books' size, the patient outcome, nursing intervention, and discharge planning sections usually do not include reference to the family or other significant people; however, the reader can assume that they are to be included along with the patient whenever appropriate.

Any undertaking of the magnitude of this series becomes the concern of many people. I specifically thank all of the very capable nursing specialists who authored or edited the individual books. Their attention to providing state-of-the-art information in a quick, usable form will provide the reader with current reference information for providing excellent patient care.

The editorial staff, particularly Patricia E. Casey and Elisabeth F. Williams, and production people at Delmar Publishers have been outstanding. Their frank criticism, comments, and encouragement have improved the quality of the series.

Finally, but most importantly, I thank my husband, John, and children, Katrina and Allison, for their sacrifices and patience during yet another publishing project.

Kathy V. Gettrust
Series Editor

LIST OF TABLES

Medical Cardiovascular Problems and Interventions

▼

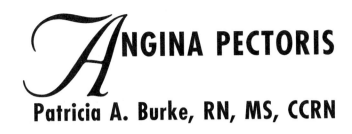

ANGINA PECTORIS

Patricia A. Burke, RN, MS, CCRN

Angina pectoris is a classic symptom of myocardial ischemia, which presents in a number of ways. Patients may describe burning, squeezing, pressure, heaviness, aching, or indigestion-like sensations in varying locations: the chest, shoulder(s), arm(s), scapulae, epigastric region, back, throat, or jaw. Precipitating factors include exertion, emotional stress, exposure to temperature extremes, or a combination thereof. Angina is frequently relieved with rest, oxygen, and/or antianginal medications. Angina may be stable (predictable in frequency and severity), unstable (new onset or worsening pain, including rest pain), or variant (unpredictable discomfort due to coronary spasm, often called Prinzmetal). If myocardial ischemia is prolonged and unrelieved, the patient is at risk for myocardial infarction. Common treatment goals include relief of pain, reduction of cardiac workload, and optimizing myocardial oxygen delivery.

ETIOLOGIES

- Coronary atherosclerosis
- Coronary spasm
- Aortic valve disease
- Hypertension
- Tachydysrhythmias if associated with coronary disease
- Congestive heart failure if associated with coronary disease
- (Less commonly, thyrotoxicosis, anemia, vasculitis)

CLINICAL MANIFESTATIONS

- Intermittent discomfort in chest, back, shoulders, scapulae, arms, throat, jaw
  - burning
  - squeezing
  - tightness or pressure
  - heaviness
  - indigestion
  - aching

- Pallor
- Diaphoresis
- Dyspnea
- Weakness
- Anxiety
- Nausea/vomiting
- Patient may clutch chest
- In elderly: dyspnea, or poorly defined throat, shoulder, or abdominal pain

CLINICAL/DIAGNOSTIC FINDINGS

- Skin—may be cool, moist
- Blood pressure—may rise or fall relative to changes in cardiac output and systemic vascular resistance
- Heart rate—may rise or fall
- Respiratory rate—may increase or decrease
- Electrocardiogram (ECG)—ischemic changes such as depressed ST segment, inverted T waves, or ventricular dysrhythmias, which normalize within several minutes after cessation of pain
- Graded exercise stress test—angina and/or ischemic ECG changes
- Cardiolite stress test—perfusion defects following exercise which are not present in resting study
- Selective coronary angiography—significant coronary arterial stenoses, or occlusion(s), and/or evidence of valvular stenoses or insufficiency. On left ventriculography, segmental wall motion defects or left ventricular hypertrophy may be present.
- Cardiac isoenzymes—are not elevated in angina pectoris
- Echocardiogram—segmental wall motion abnormalities, valvular dysfunction

NURSING DIAGNOSIS: HIGH RISK FOR DECREASED CARDIAC OUTPUT

Risk Factors
- Myocardial ischemia
- Antianginal drug-related vasodilation

Patient Outcomes
Patient will
- have vital signs within individual's normal limits.
- be awake, alert.
- make postural changes without orthostatic hypotension.
- have warm, dry skin.

- have urine output of 30 mL/hr or more.
- have peripheral pulses of individual's usual quality.

Nursing Interventions	**Rationales**
Administer antianginal agents as prescribed; monitor patient for hypotension and hypertension before, during, and after administration. See Table 1.1.	Hypotension is an indicator of falling cardiac output, which may worsen myocardial ischemia. Hypertension, because it involves increased systemic vascular resistance and increased left ventricular workload, will increase myocardial oxygen demand and aggravate angina. While nitrates, morphine, beta blockers, and calcium channel blockers are all drugs of choice to reduce myocardial oxygen consumption, they alter heart rate, contractility, venous return to the heart, and systemic vascular resistance. All must be titrated carefully to avoid undesirable degrees of hypotension.
Ensure patent intravenous (IV) line.	For rapid systemic effect, many antianginals and analgesics such as nitrates and morphine are given intravenously.

NURSING DIAGNOSIS: HIGH RISK FOR ALTERED TISSUE PERFUSION—CENTRAL AND PERIPHERAL

Risk Factors
- Decreased cardiac output
- Myocardial oxygen supply-demand imbalance

Patient Outcomes
Patient will
- have vital signs within individual's normal limits.
- palpable peripheral pulses of usual quality.
- have warm, dry skin
- exhibit pink skin undertones and mucous membranes
- Verbalize that he or she is comfortable.
- have normal ECG as compared to baseline, without ischemic changes.

Table 1.1 • Antianginal Drugs

Category	Therapeutic Features	Side Effects and Considerations
NITRATES include such agents as IV nitroglycerin, sublingual nitroglycerin tablets and spray, oral nitroglycerin, and transdermal nitroglycerin.	Nitrates relax smooth muscle, causing venodilation. The resulting venous pooling of blood decreases preload and reduces myocardial oxygen demand. Nitrates also dilate coronary arteries and transiently improve oxygenation and blood flow to the myocardium. Sublingual and IV routes are preferred for rapid anginal relief. A typical sublingual nitroglycerin dose is 0.4–0.6 mg and can be repeated every 5 min for three consecutive tablets. Patients will usually exhibit relief after one to three tablets. Nitroglycerin can be taken prophylactically prior to angina-provoking activities. If no relief, other therapeutic modalities should be considered. Intravenous nitroglycerin is titrated in micrograms per minute and must be run via infusion pump. It is usually started at 5 μg/min and titrated to the lowest dose that relieves pain.	Nitrates can rapidly lower blood pressure, necessitating an adequate means of monitoring the patient. Consideration should be given to arterial monitoring for the patient on IV nitroglycerin. Because of the affinity of nitroglycerin for plastic IV bags and tubing, special nonabsorbable administration sets must be used. Intravenous nitroglycerin must not be stopped abruptly unless the patient develops profound hypotension or the patient may have rebound ischemia. All forms of nitroglycerin can produce headache, hypotension, nausea, diaphoresis, tachy- and bradyarrhythmias, and in some cases, tolerance.

Table 1.1 • Continued

Category	Therapeutic Features	Side Effects and Considerations
BETA BLOCKERS include such agents as propranolol, labetalol, esmolol, pindolol, and nadolol.	Beta blockers are given orally or intravenously, in doses specific to the agent given. They block beta-adrenergic stimulation of the heart, resulting in negative inotropic and chronotropic effects: heart rate slows, and atrioventricular (AV) nodal conduction time is prolonged. Blood pressure is thus decreased, diastolic filling time is prolonged, and myocardial oxygen demand decreases.	Beta blockers must be used carefully in patients with decreased left ventricular function, as they can precipitate heart failure. Heart rate must be assessed, and the drug should be stopped if it causes persistent sinus bradycardia or progressive heart block. Asthmatics and others prone to bronchospasm tolerate beta blockers poorly; wheezing is an indication to stop the drug. Patients should be instructed not to abruptly stop beta blockers without medical supervision, as rebound angina and hypertension can occur.
CALCIUM CHANNEL BLOCKERS include such drugs as diltiazem, nifedipine, nicardipine, isradipine, and verapamil. Nifedipine and diltiazem are most commonly used for angina management.	Calcium channel blockers decrease slow calcium current in the AV junction, lengthening its refractory time. They slow calcium movement into arteriolar smooth muscle and thus decrease systemic vascular resistance, afterload, and blood pressure. Coronary blood flow and oxygenation improve, and myocardial oxygen demand diminishes. For angina, calcium channel blockers can be given sublingually and orally in doses specific to the agent.	Headache, flushing, and dizziness can all be results of vasodilatation. Gastrointestinal distress, bradycardia, hypotension, and conduction disturbances are also possible side effects. Intravenous agents should be given in a setting where cardiac monitoring and intensive medical support is available.

▼

Nursing Interventions	Rationales
Have patient stop any activity and either sit or lie down.	Decreasing skeletal muscle work reduces oxygen demand on myocardium.
Obtain and assess 12–lead ECG for signs of myocardial ischemia.	In new-onset or unstable angina, ECG can be particularly helpful in determining the degree and location of ischemia and in evaluating relief measures. During repeated pain episodes, it is important to consider whether the ECG will yield any new information. Repetitive ECGs for random episodes of angina delay treatment measures.
Assess and record patient's color, skin temperature, and peripheral pulses.	Comparing these observations with baseline measurements can be helpful in determining peripheral perfusion. Cool extremities and thready peripheral pulses are indicative of poor peripheral perfusion and low or falling cardiac output.

NURSING DIAGNOSIS: HIGH RISK FOR IMPAIRED GAS EXCHANGE

Risk Factors
- Splinting from pain
- Subjective dyspnea
- Associated heart failure

Patient Outcomes
Patient will
- exhibit normal rate and quality of respirations.
- verbalize ability to relax and rest.
- exhibit lungs clear to auscultation.
- exhibit pulse oximetry 92% or greater.

Nursing Interventions	Rationales
Place patient in semi-Fowler's position.	Elevating head of bed assists patient with diaphragmatic excursion.
Administer oxygen per unit standards, usually 2–6 L/min per nasal cannula.	Supplemental oxygen enhances oxygen delivery to myocardial and peripheral tissues. Subjectively, it may relieve the dyspneic patient.
Monitor pulse oximetry and adjust O_2 to maintain pulse oximetry 92% or greater.	
Assess and document lung sounds on a routine basis.	The presence of rales indicates fluid accumulation in the alveolar-capillary membranes, which will impede oxygen and carbon dioxide exchange. Rales may also indicate heart failure, a condition to which many patients with coronary artery disease are prone.

NURSING DIAGNOSIS: ACUTE PAIN

Related To myocardial tissue hypoxia and/or muscle spasm

Defining Characteristics
Agitation, restlessnesss
Patient verbalizes pain
Nonverbal signs of pain, such as grimace, muscle tension, self-focusing
Diaphoresis
Blood pressure and pulse changes

Patient Outcomes
- Patient can describe intensity and nature of pain.
- Pain episodes are promptly treated and resolved.
- Nonverbal pain cues are absent.
- Patient verbalizes confidence in ability to promptly obtain help.
- Patient verbalizes understanding of anginal mechanism.
- Patient verbalizes understanding of methods of prevention/relief of anginal episodes.

Nursing Interventions	Rationales
Respond consistently and promptly to patient summons with pain-relieving measures.	Quick nursing action enhances patient confidence, gives patient sense of being able to control outcomes, and decreases stress and uncertainty.
Discuss causes of angina with patient and methods of prevention/relief of episodes. Plan realistically daily schedule with patient, clustering activities and providing for periods of rest.	Perceived lack of control, coupled with lack of knowledge, makes hospitalization difficult for most patients. Agreed-upon goals of care and treatment plans that are shared with the patient enhance patient comfort and well-being, and promote open communication between nurse and patient.
Teach patient actions and side effects of antianginal medications.	Detailed knowledge related to these agents enhances safe and effective care.

DISCHARGE PLANNING/CONTINUITY OF CARE

- Assess patient's understanding of angina, including precipitating factors, treatment, and follow-up, and reinforce knowledge and problem solving as necessary.
- Ensure that patient has and understands medication, diet, and activity instructions.
- Facilitate follow-up visit with physician.

REFERENCES

Alspach, J. G. (Ed.). (1991). *Core curriculum for critical care nursing.* Philadelphia: Saunders.

Eberts, M. A. (1986). Advances in the management of angina pectoris. *Journal of Cardiovascular Nursing, 1*(1), 15–29.

Ford, R. D. (Ed.). (1986). *Cardiovascular care handbook.* Springhouse, PA: Springhouse Corporation.

Murphy, T. G., & Bennett, E. J. (1992). Low-tech, high touch perfusion assessment. *American Journal of Nursing, 92*(5), 36–48.

Thompson, L., Wood, C., & Wallhagen, M. (1992). Geriatric acute myocardial infarction: A challenge to recognition, prompt diagnosis, and appropriate care. *Critical Care Nursing Clinics of North America, 4,* 291–300.

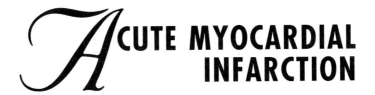ACUTE MYOCARDIAL INFARCTION

Mary G. Schigoda, RN, MSN, CCRN

Acute myocardial infarction (AMI) is a process which results in the death of myocardial muscle. It occurs during myocardial ischemia that is of sufficient intensity and duration to produce recognizable necrosis of the myocardial tissue. It is usually preceded by atherosclerosis and decreased blood flow, which leads to ischemia, injury, and ultimately, death of a portion of the myocardium.

ETIOLOGIES

Sustained myocardial ischemia, resulting in irreversible cell damage and death. This may be precipitated by
- Coronary thrombus
- Coronary spasm
- Emboli
- Hemorrhage
- Atherosclerosis

CLINICAL MANIFESTATIONS

- Severe, persistent chest pain
- Anxiety
- Nausea/vomiting
- Diaphoresis
- Shortness of breath (SOB)

CLINICAL/DIAGNOSTIC FINDINGS

- Electrocardiogram (ECG)
  - ischemia, injury, and/or infarct patterns
  - evolutionary phases of the infarct

- location of transmural (Q-wave) infarct
- dysrhythmias/conduction disturbances
- left ventricular (LV) aneurysm formation
- atrial/ventricular enlargement

- Chest x-ray (CXR):congestive heart failure (CHF)
- Radionuclide studies
  - thallium-201 scanning:differentiates ischemic from normal or infarcted muscle
  - technetium-99m pyrophosphate isotope scanning:identifies area of infarction
- Echocardiogram (ECHO):identifies abnormal ventricular wall motion and mechanical complications of AMI (i.e., papillary muscle dysfunction/rupture)
- Cardiac catheterization and angiography:identifies stenotic/occluded coronary arteries
- Cardiac enzyme levels
  - CK (creatine kinase) elevated
  - CK-MB (CK isoenzyme) elevated
  - LDH (lactase dehydrogenase) elevated
  - LDH-1 (LDH isoenzyme) elevated
  - LDH-2 (LDH isoenzyme) elevated (all due to myocardial muscle necrosis)
- ESR (erythrocyte sedimentation rate) increased
- WBC (white blood cell) count increased (both due to inflammatory response)

NURSING DIAGNOSIS: ACUTE PAIN

Related To inadequate myocardial perfusion and systemic response to AMI

Defining Characteristics

Agitation and restlessness
Alteration in muscle tone (ranging from listlessness to rigidity)
Autonomic responses (diaphoresis, blood pressure and heart rate changes, pupillary dilation, increased or decreased respiratory rate)
Distraction behavior (moaning, crying)
Facial expressions of pain (grimacing, dull eyes, flat affect, twitching)
Guarding behavior and splinting of pain site
Inability to concentrate
Irritability
Narrowed focus (altered time perception, impaired thought process, withdrawal from social contact)
Self-focus

Patient Outcomes

Patient will
- report and describe pain.
- report relief of pain.
- not demonstrate complications from therapeutic interventions.

Nursing Interventions	Rationales
Assess pain promptly, noting verbal complaints, nonverbal clues, and hemodynamic response. Note location, duration, intensity, quality, and radiation.	Because pain is a subjective experience, the descriptions and appearance of patients in pain may vary greatly. A delay in reporting pain may hinder pain relief, requiring increased amounts of medication. Severe pain also stimulates the sympathetic nervous system (SNS), resulting in catecholamine release and increased oxygen consumption.
Institute measures to relieve ischemic pain in a safe and timely manner per physician prescription or unit protocol, including: 1. Administer IV analgesics.	Analgesics, such as morphine sulfate, reduce pain, provide sedation, and reduce myocardial workload.
2. Administer antianginal medications.	Antianginal medications, such as nitrates, beta blockers, and calcium antagonists, relieve pain by enhancing oxygen supply and reducing myocardial work and oxygen demand.
3. Instruct on relaxation techniques, such as guided imagery.	These techniques may provide pain relief through distraction, giving the patient a sense of control over the situation.
Monitor vital signs before and after the administration of pain medications.	Hypotension and/or respiratory depression may occur as a result of narcotic administration.

Nursing Interventions	Rationales
Institute measures to decrease myocardial workload:	
1. Promote rest through the provision of physical comfort, freedom from worry, and sufficient sleep.	Rest reduces myocardial work and oxygen consumption, thus limiting the risk of infarct extension and further reduction in cardiac output (CO).
2. Provide small, easily digested meals. Progress diet, starting with clear liquids, as tolerated.	Large meals may increase myocardial work and oxygen consumption. Gastric motility also may be decreased from the administration of narcotics for pain relief, resulting in nausea. Clear liquids are provided to decrease risk of aspiration in case of cardiac arrest.
3. Restrict caffeine (coffee, tea, and cola) intake.	Caffeine is a cardiac stimulant, which increases heart rate. In light of reduced oxygen supply, this may precipitate pain from ischemia. Observe for withdrawal symptoms in patients with excessive prior intake. Gradual reduction may be preferred.
Institute measures to improve myocardial perfusion in a safe and timely manner per physician prescription or unit protocol, including:	
1. Administer supplemental oxygen.	Hypoxemia is common in patients with AMI. To prevent an increase in systemic vascular resistance (SVR) and a decrease in CO, oxygen should only be used when arterial oxygen saturation determinations indicate a hypoxemic state exists.

Nursing Interventions	**Rationales**
2. Administer thrombolytic therapy.	Thrombolytic therapy improves coronary blood flow by lysing (dissolving) thrombus that occludes coronary arteries. It is often effective in reperfusing reversibly injured myocardium, thus reducing infarct size, LV dysfunction, and mortality. (Refer to Thrombolytic Therapy.)
3. Prepare for percutaneous transluminal coronary angioplasty (PTCA).	Percutaneous transluminal coronary angioplasty can be used to achieve reperfusion, and is used when thrombolytic therapy is contraindicated or unsuccessful or when severe stenosis remains following successful thrombolysis. (Refer to Percutaneous Transluminal Coronary Angioplasty.)
4. Prepare for surgical myocardial revascularization (MR), if indicated.	Surgical revascularization can improve myocardial oxygenation and limit infarct size. Although it appears effective if carried out within 4 hr of AMI onset, it is logistically very difficult to accomplish unless the patient is already in the hospital awaiting surgery. (Refer to Cardiac Surgery.)
Assess for nausea, vomiting, and hiccuping; administer prescribed medications if needed.	Nausea and vomiting are initially caused by the systemic stress response to AMI. Later analgesics and other cardiac drugs or decreased perfusion to the gastrointestinal (GI) tract may cause nausea and vomiting. Hiccuping often accompanies inferior wall MI, and is caused by diaphragmatic stimulation from the inflamed inferior myocardial surface. Vagal stimulation resulting from the Valsalva maneuver during vomiting can provoke dysrhythmias.

Nursing Interventions	Rationales
Assess for bladder distention.	Bladder distention is a problem in men with prostatic hypertrophy. It is aggravated by medications, such as atropine, sedatives, and opiates, as well as by bedrest.
Assess for pericardial pain, pericardial friction rub, and cardiac tamponade.	Pericarditis is an inflammatory process that develops in about 10–15% of AMI patients 2–7 days postinfarct.
Pain is usually aggravated by deep inspiration and lessened by leaning forward while sitting.	Transient pericardial friction rubs are common in the first 48 hr. Pericarditis is a relative contraindication for anticoagulant or thrombolytic therapy because of the risk of hemorrhage and pericardial tamponade (Refer to Cardiac Tamponade).
Administer prescribed anti-inflammatory and analgesic medications to relieve pain if indicated.	Aspirin, indomethacin, or corticosteroids may be prescribed to reduce inflammation and pain.
Assess for signs/symptoms of Dressler's syndrome, including fever, pleuro/pericardial chest pain, pericardial friction rub, and pleural effusion. Administer aspirin, nonsteroidal anti-inflammatory drugs (NSAIDs), and/or analgesics.	Dressler's syndrome (post–myocardial infarction syndrome) is an uncommon complication that develops 1–2 weeks after AMI. The most widely accepted cause is an autoimmune response, although a viral etiology has been proposed. These medications are most useful in relieving the discomfort associated with Dressler's syndrome.
Promote rest, provide reassurance, and encourage relaxation exercises.	These interventions reduce the anxiety typically seen with Dressler's syndrome.

NURSING DIAGNOSIS: DECREASED CARDIAC OUTPUT

Related To
- Electrical factors (rate, rhythm, conduction disturbances)
- Mechanical factors (altered preload, afterload, contractility)
- Structural factors (papillary muscle dysfunction, ventricular septum rupture, ventricular aneurysm, ventricular rupture)

Defining Characteristics

Abnormal arterial blood gases
Abnormal CXR
Abnormal heart sounds (S_3 and S_4)
Abnormal hemoglobin and hematocrit
Angina
Cough
Cyanosis; pallor of skin and mucous membranes
Crackles
Decreased activity tolerance
Decreased peripheral pulses
Dyspnea
Dysrhythmias; electrocardiographic changes
Edema (peripheral and/or pulmonary)
Ejection fraction (EF) < 40%
Elevated cardiac enzymes
Fatigue
Jugular venous distention (JVD)
Oliguria; anuria
Orthopnea
Paroxysmal nocturnal dyspnea (PND)
Shortness of breath (SOB)
Variations in blood pressure readings
Variations in hemodynamic readings
Weakness
Weight gain

Other Defining Characteristics

Abdominal distention
Anorexia
Ascites
Change in mental state/level of consciousness (LOC)
Diaphoresis
Anxiety
Frothy sputum
Left parasternal lift
Palpitations

Patient Outcomes

Patient will
- demonstrate hemodynamic stability and optimal cardiac output.
- maintain optimal heart rate and rhythm without conduction disturbance (electrical factors).
- respond appropriately to the prescribed treatment if a rate, rhythm, or conduction disturbance occurs.
- maintain optimal preload, afterload, and contractility (mechanical factors).

- respond positively to therapies to maintain preload, afterload, and contractility.
- not demonstrate papillary muscle rupture/dysfunction, ventricular septal defect, ventricular aneurysm, or ventricular rupture (structural factors).
- respond appropriately to corrective therapy if structural complications occur.
- not demonstrate complications of hemodynamic monitoring or other diagnostic tests and procedures.
- not demonstrate signs/symptoms of cardiogenic shock.

Nursing Interventions	Rationales
Assess vital signs.	Hypotension is fairly common and may result from hypoperfusion, vagal stimulation, dysrhythmias, pain, anxiety, catecholamine release.
Auscultate heart sounds, noting 1. S_1 and S_2	Normal heart sounds are frequently muffled during the acute phase of a MI.
2. S_3 and S_4	Abnormal heart sounds, such as S_3 and S_4, are indicative of early cardiac decompensation. Usually S_3 is associated with CHF, whereas S_4 is usually associated with myocardial ischemia, loss of ventricular compliance, and systemic/pulmonic hypertension.
3. Murmurs	Murmurs are due to turbulent blood flow through an incompetent valve or septal defect.
4. Rubs	Presence of a rub with AMI is associated with pericarditis or pericardial effusion.
Auscultate breath sounds.	Crackles may develop, reflecting pulmonary congestion.
Assess hemodynamic parameters, noting mean arterial pressure (MAP), pulmonary artery pressure (PAP), pulmonary capillary wedge pressure (PCWP), systemic vascular resistance (SVR), cardiac output/cardiac index (CO/CI).	Accurate measurement of ventricular function and vascular responses is useful in managing therapeutic interventions, evaluating activity tolerance, and detecting complications of AMI. (Refer to Congestive Heart Failure and Cardiogenic Shock.)

Nursing Interventions	Rationales
Monitor intake and output (I&O) and daily weight.	Recording I&O over a 24-hr period identifies trends in fluid balance. Weight increases with volume overload and pulmonary congestion.
Monitor for rate, rhythm, and conduction disturbances: 1. tachycardia	Tachycardia occurs in response to decreased vagal tone or sympathetic nervous system activation with resultant catecholamine release. Sustained tachycardia may aggravate ischemia as it shortens diastolic filling time (decreasing coronary artery perfusion) and increases oxygen demand.
2. bradycardia	Bradycardia occurs in response to a decrease in blood flow to the sinus node or as a result of excessive parasympathetic activity.
3. conduction disturbances	Conduction problems occur as a result of reduced oxygen supply to the sinoatrial (SA) and atrioventricular (AV) nodes and the infarct itself, which may extend into the conduction tissue.
4. ventricular dysrhythmias	Ventricular dysrhythmias are common following AMI. Ischemia causes ventricular irritability which may culminate in life-threatening ventricular tachycardia or fibrillation.
Institute measures to manage dysrhythmias per physician prescription or unit protocol, including 1. antidysrhythmic medications (see Table 2.1)	Dysrhythmias may lower stroke volume (SV), thereby reducing CO.

Nursing Interventions	**Rationales**
2. insertion/maintenance of temporary cardiac pacing	Cardiac pacing may be necessary as a temporary support in the acute phase of the MI. A permanently implanted pacemaker may be required if the infarct has severely damaged the conduction system. (Refer to Artificial Cardiac Pacing.)
3. cardioversion/defibrillation/ implementation of other emergency interventions	Sudden coronary occlusion, infarct extension, and/or lethal dysrhythmias may precipitate cardiac arrest and require immediate life-saving interventions.
Assess for mechanical dysfunction, including 1. hypotension	Labile blood pressure or orthostatic hypotension may reflect hypovolemia.
2. SOB, dyspnea, orthopnea, S_3, pulmonary crackles	Shortness of breath, dyspnea, orthopnea, S_3, and pulmonary crackles reflect left-sided volume overload and pulmonary congestion.
3. JVD, hepatic engorgement, peripheral edema	Jugular venous distention, hepatic engorgement, and peripheral edema reflect increasing cardiac decompensation. Right-sided volume overload leading to systemic venous congestion may result from the progression of left-sided heart failure or from right ventricular (RV) infarction.
4. invasive hemodynamic monitoring techniques (arterial, pulmonary artery, CO catheters)	Invasive hemodynamic monitoring aids in the early recognition of complications associated with AMI and assists with determinations of cardiac function and response to pharmacological and mechanical interventions.

Nursing Interventions	**Rationales**
Maintain mechanical function by administering (per physician prescription or unit protocol): 1. supplemental oxygen 2. IV fluids	Intravenous fluids need to be administered cautiously, as an inadvertent bolus of fluid may result in pulmonary congestion and further cardiac decompensation.
3. diuretics, vasodilators, inotropic agents	Cardiac output may be improved by combinations of (1) diuretics to prevent/correct volume overload (preload), (2) vasodilators to decrease SVR (afterload), and (3) inotropic agents to enhance contractility.
4. intra-aortic balloon pump (IABP) therapy	The IABP counterpulsation provides systolic unloading and diastolic augmentation, decreasing the work of the heart and enhancing coronary artery perfusion.
Assess for structural dysfunction: 1. papillary muscle dysfunction/rupture—systolic murmur, left-sided heart failure, pulmonary edema	Papillary muscle dysfunction causes mitral valve insufficiency/regurgitation with backflow of blood into the pulmonary system, resulting in pulmonary congestion. With papillary muscle rupture, the patient is most likely to have an acute onset of CHF associated with dysrhythmias, cyanosis, and apprehension. Without aggressive management, death will most likely occur within hours or days.
2. ventricular septum rupture—pansystolic murmur, heart failure, hypotension	Ventricular septum rupture occurs in 1–3% of AMI patients and is most common in the first week after AMI. Depending on the size of the defect, CHF or cardiogenic shock ensues, as left-to-right shunting of blood results.

Nursing Interventions	**Rationales**
3. ventricular aneurysm—persistent S₃ gallop, heart failure, dysrhythmias, and activity intolerance. Ventricular aneurysm develops in 12–15% of patients who survive AMI.	It may involve an area of the ventricle which is akinetic (not moving at all) or dyskinetic (expanding rather than contracting) during systole. Much of the ventricle's pumping force is lost due to ischemic or nonfunctional cardiac muscle. Complications include CHF, mural thrombus formation and potential embolization, and ventricular dysrhythmias.
4. ventricular rupture—electromechanical dissociation (EMD), intractable heart failure, cardiogenic shock, death	Ventricular rupture accounts for 10% of the deaths related to AMI. With rupture of the free wall of the ventricle, cardiac tamponade occurs, rapidly compressing the heart and inhibiting ventricular ejection. Cardiac arrest and death usually follow in rapid succession.
Monitor for early signs/symptoms of cardiogenic shock: hypotension (systolic pressure < 90 mmHg), tachycardia, oliguria, poor peripheral perfusion, decreased level of consciousness).	Cardiogenic shock develops in 10–20% of patients hospitalized with AMI. It occurs when 40% or more of the LV muscle mass is lost, which is accompanied by a marked reduction in CO and overall inadequate tissue perfusion.
Institute measures to manage cardiogenic shock per physician prescription or unit protocol, including 1. pharmacological support (inotropic agents, vasodilators, diuretics)	

Nursing Interventions	**Rationales**
2. mechanical support [IABP, ventricular assist device VAD)]	Management of cardiogenic shock is aimed at improving myocardial contractility without increasing myocardial work, raising arterial pressure to maintain adequate coronary perfusion, and lowering peripheral vascular resistance without compromising renal blood flow. (Refer to Cardiogenic Shock and Ventricular Assist Devices.)

Table 2.1 • Antidysrhythmic Drug Classification

Class	Effect
Class I Ia. Quinidine, procainamide, disopyramide, phenytoin Ib. Mexiletine, tocainide, lidocaine, lorcainide Ic. Encainide, flecainide	These agents depress the maximal rate of depolarization of the cardiac action potential. These drugs have local anesthetic properties that affect nerve and myocardial membranes and inhibit the early rapid influx of sodium into the cell during the rapid upstroke phase of the action potential.
Class II Propranolol, metoprolol, atenolol, timolol	These agents include the β-adrenergic blocking drugs, which block the sympathetic nervous system's dysrhythmogenic effects on the myocardium and thus depress phase 4 depolarization of the cardiac action potential.
Class III Bretylium, amiodarone	These agents lengthen the absolute refractory period and prolong the duration of the action potential.
Class IV Verapamil, diltiazem	These agents inhibit the influx of extracellular calcium through the slow calcium channels during phase 2 of the cardiac action potential.

NURSING DIAGNOSIS: HIGH RISK FOR ALTERED TISSUE PERFUSION—PERIPHERAL

Risk Factors
- Atherosclerosis
- Disruption of arterial flow (e.g., acute thrombosis)
- Disruption of venous flow (e.g., thrombophlebitis)
- Hypervolemia (e.g., CHF, renal failure)
- Hypovolemia (e.g., dehydration)
- Inadequate circulation (e.g., immobility)
- Invasive lines (e.g., hemodynamic lines, IABP)
- Medications (e.g., vasoactive drugs)
- Obstruction (e.g., edema)
- Reduced arterial flow (e.g., hypertension)
- Reduced venous flow (e.g., varicosities)
- Spasm (e.g., Raynaud's disease)
- Vasoconstriction (e.g., stress, smoking)
- Ventilation/perfusion disorders (e.g., pulmonary
- emboli)

Patient Outcomes
Patient will be free of signs/symptoms of arterial/venous thrombus/embolus formation.

Nursing Interventions	Rationales
Assess for diminished/absent bowel sounds, abdominal distention/pain, constipation, and fecal impaction	The vasoconstrictive response associated with decreased perfusion to the mesentery can produce abdominal pain/nausea and loss of peristalsis, leading to ileus. This may be aggravated by the use of narcotics, bedrest, decreased roughage in the diet, and potassium depletion after diuresis
Assess for signs and symptoms of peripheral and pulmonary embolism, including: 1. changes in peripheral pulses (especially in cannulated extremities)	Deep venous thrombosis (DVT) occurs in about 30% and arterial emboli in about 5% of patients with AMI. Vasoconstriction results in decreased tissue perfusion.

Nursing Interventions	Rationales
2. pallor, cyanosis, mottling, cool, clammy skin	Localized occurrence of these signs may indicate the presence of peripheral embolus/thrombus resulting from the cellular damage occurring with decreased tissue perfusion.
3. Homan's sign (pain in calf on dorsiflexion), erythema, edema	These are indicators of thrombophlebitis.
4. sudden onset of dyspnea, with/ without chest pain, feelings of impending doom	These are indicators of pulmonary emboli resulting from a sudden reduction in gas exchange.
Apply antiembolic hose, removing at least once per shift.	Antiembolic hose limit venous stasis, improve venous return, and reduce risk of thrombophlebitis in the patient on bedrest. Removal once per shift allows for inspection of lower extremities and assessment of peripheral pulses.
Do passive leg exercises (avoiding isometric exercises).	Passive leg exercises enhance venous return. Isometric exercises increase myocardial oxygen consumption and may adversely affect CO.
Administer prescribed anticoagulant/antiplatelet medications.	Low-dose heparin may be given prophylactically in high-risk patients (atrial fibrillation, ventricular aneurysm, cardiogenic shock, and history of thrombophlebitis) to reduce risk of thrombophlebitis or mural thrombus formation. Heparin also is used following thrombolytic therapy to prevent recurrent thrombus formation. The antiplatelet effects of aspirin have been shown to prevent thrombus formation and thus AMI.

NURSING DIAGNOSIS: ANXIETY

Related To pathophysiological, situational, and treatment-related factors

Defining Characteristics
Anger
Change in appetite
Change in sleep patterns
Chest tightness
Crying
Difficulty in expressing self
Distractable
Facial/muscle tension
Hyperventilation
Indecisive
Irritable
Palpitations
Selective inattention
Tachycardia
Trembling
Verbalizes/demonstrates inability to concentrate
Withdrawal

Patient Outcomes
Patient/family will
- express anxiety, fears, and concerns.
- demonstrate reduced levels of anxiety and not experience severe anxiety/panic.
- institute effective coping behaviors.
- not demonstrate increased anxiety levels on transfer or discharge.
- verbalize and demonstrate acceptance of changed life situation.

Nursing Interventions	Rationales
Assess for anxiety, fears, concerns, and coping in patient and family.	Acute myocardial infarction is an unexpected, life-threatening event with an uncertain outcome. It may disrupt and change family roles and relationships.
Institute measures to reduce anxiety, including:	Anxiety, especially severe anxiety, may precipitate or aggravate chest pain by increasing myocardial oxygen consumption, worsening ischemia. This may potentiate complications, such as dysrhythmias.
1. explanation of illness, coronary care unit (CCU) environment, therapeutic regime	Patient and family are in an unfamiliar environment. Patient also is being subjected to multiple procedures/treatments while experiencing severe pain.

Nursing Interventions	Rationales
2. decrease in sensory stimulation	This intervention enhances rest and ability to cope effectively.
3. guiding patient and family in the use of relaxation techniques, imagery, music	These techniques may reduce distress and impart a sense of control over the situation.
Administer prescribed medications, as needed, including narcotic analgesics and sedative/hypnotic agents.	Anxiety may contribute to ongoing ischemic pain. Ongoing anxiety related to the losses precipitated by the MI may be present in varying degrees for some time.
Recognize and accept anxiety, denial, anger, depression, and aggressive sexual behavior as coping behaviors. Provide emotion- and problem-focused support.	Coping behaviors may be used to lessen the emotional distress or manage the problem. Emotion-focused behaviors include denial, repression, displacement, projection, rationalization, and paranoid reactions. They are common and may be beneficial, particularly during the acute phase of the MI. Problem-focused behaviors include strategies such as defining the problem, gathering information, weighing alternative solutions, and determining appropriate action. Both types of behaviors should be encouraged and supported.
Provide structured teaching before transfer and discharge.	Anxiety associated with transfer and discharge can be viewed as a special form of separation anxiety, a break from the security of constant observation. Pretransfer and predischarge teaching can significantly reduce the patient's and family's level of anxiety.

Nursing Interventions	Rationales
Assess patient's and family's usual roles, discuss feelings about changes in role performance, and facilitate family function, by 1. permitting flexible visiting, whenever possible 2. encouraging family to participate in care, if they and patient wish 3. allowing private family time daily. 4. referring to cardiac rehabilitation program	The majority of issues are related to role surface after hospitalization, as the family learns to live together once again. Referral to cardiac rehabilitation while still in the hospital, with continuation in the program after discharge, can be very beneficial in assisting with the problems that then arise. These other interventions can facilitate the maintenance of family relationships while in the hospital.

NURSING DIAGNOSIS: KNOWLEDGE DEFICIT

Related To myocardial infarction and its implications for lifestyle changes

Defining Characteristics
Inaccurate follow-through of instructions
Inadequate performance of a skill
Inappropriate or exaggerated behaviors, e.g., agitated, apathetic, hostile, hysterical
Lack of recall
Verbalizations indicating inadequate understanding, misinterpretation, or misconception of desired health behavior

Patient Outcomes
Patient and family will verbalize/demonstrate understanding of self-care following AMI, angina versus infarction, CAD risk factor modification, medications, activity progression, and relaxation strategies.

Nursing Interventions	Rationales
Assess needs and teach appropriate content regarding: 1. self-care following AMI 2. signs/symptoms of angina versus infarction 3. CAD risk factor modification 4. medications 5. activity progression (including sexual activities) 6. relaxation strategies	Effective teaching takes into account patient/family readiness to learn, preexisting knowledge, phase of recovery from illness, and major concerns.

DISCHARGE PLANNING/CONTINUITY OF CARE

- Provide structured pretransfer teaching, including overview of the new environment (targeted length of stay, expected nurse/patient ratios, targeted progress), stress management techniques, and an explanation that transfer or discharge is a sign of progress.
- Inform patient that after transfer telemetry monitoring will continue for about 3–5 days, cardiac rehabilitation will be introduced, and feelings of anxiety or depression are normal.
- Instruct the patient to report any chest pain, or shortness of breath.
- Provide structured predischarge teaching (see Knowledge Deficit).

REFERENCES

Gawlinski, A. (1989). Nursing care after AMI: A comprehensive review. *Critical Care Nursing Quarterly, 12*(2), 64–72.

Gettrust, K. V., & Brabec, P. D. (1992). *Nursing diagnosis in clinical practice*. Albany, NY: Delmar.

Haak, S. W., & Huether, S. E. (1992). The person with myocardial infarction. In C. E. Guzetta & B. M. Dossey (Eds.), *Cardiovascular nursing—Holistic practice* (pp. 252–298). St. Louis, MO: Mosby Year Book.

Mayberry-Toth, B., & Landron, S. (1989). Complications associated with acute myocardial infarction. *Critical Care Nursing Quarterly, 12*(2), 49–63.

Moorhouse, M. S., Geissler, A. C., & Doenges, M. E., (1987). *Critical care plans*, Philadelphia: Davis.

Riegel, B. (1988). Acute myocardial infarction: Nursing interventions to optimize oxygen supply and demand. In L. Kern (Ed.), *Cardiac critical care nursing* (pp. 59–90). Rockville, MD: Aspen.

Toth, J. C. (1980). Effect of structured preparation for transfer on patient anxiety on leaving the coronary care unit. *Nursing Research, 29*, 28.

▼

*J*HROMBOLYTIC THERAPY

Alice T. Kramer, RN, BSN, MS, CEN

Thrombolytic therapy is a pharmacological strategy that intervenes with the natural process of an acute myocardial infarction (AMI), permitting the salvage of myocardial muscle which would otherwise have been irreversibly damaged. The presence of atherosclerosis is the underlying basis for the events that lead to most AMIs. Over time, the plaque impedes blood flow within the artery, vasoactive substances are released, and a thrombus is formed. Thrombolytic therapy induces pharmacological dissolution of the thrombus in the coronary artery by conversion of plasminogen to plasmin. The plasmin degrades the insoluble fibrin strands and the clot dissolves. The clinical benefits of thrombolytic therapy in AMI patients are a reduction of myocardial infarct size, preservation of left ventricular function, decreased incidence of congestive heart failure (CHF), and reduction of patient mortality.

ETIOLOGIES (AMENABLE TO THROMBOLYTIC THERAPY)

- Underlying atherosclerosis
- Platelet aggregation
- Coronary artery thrombosis

CLINICAL MANIFESTATIONS

Acute Myocardial Infarction
- Chest pain—typically more severe and prolonged than angina and most often unrelieved by nitroglycerin
- Radiation or localization of pain to the neck, jaw, back, shoulder, substernal region, left arm, or epigastric area
- Diaphoresis
- Pale/gray color
- Restlessness
- Nausea, vomiting

- Alterations in blood pressure, heart rate/rhythm, and respirations depending on the location of infarct and extent of myocardium involved
- S_4 and/or S_3 heart sounds depending on the extent of reduced left ventricular compliance (see acute MI care plan for more specifics)

CLINICAL/DIAGNOSTIC FINDINGS PRIOR TO THROMBOLYTIC THERAPY

- Characteristic ECG changes that may include abnormal, persistent Q waves, elevation of the ST segment, and symmetrical inversion of the T wave

Reperfusion of occluded coronary artery after thrombolytic therapy
- Resolution of ST-segment elevation as noted on ECG
- Development of dysrhythmias such as premature ventricular contractions (PVCs), ventricular tachycardia, accelerated idioventricular rhythms, sinus bradycardia, or AV blocks
- Coronary angiography: Direct visualization of affected artery will verify lysis of thrombus and diagnose extent of remaining occlusion and/or stenosis
- Thallium scan and stress test—used to identify perfusion defects which reflect infarcted tissue
- Multigated blood pool imaging (MUGA) scan and echocardiography (ECHO)—helpful in identifying wall motion abnormalities and decreased ejection fractions

NURSING DIAGNOSIS: ACUTE CHEST PAIN

Related To
- Occluded coronary artery
- Myocardial ischemia
- Delay in diagnosis and treatment of AMI

Defining Characteristics

Abrupt onset, usually occurring at rest or without provocation
Generally constant and cannot be reproduced by palpation or change in position
Often indicated by bringing clenched fist to sternum or by pointing to anterior chest surface
Described as crushing or viselike
May radiate to arm(s), neck, jaw, epigastrium
Unrelieved by rest or medications taken at home

Patient Outcomes

Patient will

- experience relief of ischemic myocardial chest pain and associated symptoms.
- receive prompt diagnosis of AMI and evaluation for the appropriateness of thrombolytic therapy.
- experience reperfusion of the occluded coronary artery, as clinically evidenced by
  - resolution of ST-segment elevation
  - development of dysrhythmias
  - relief of chest pain

Nursing Interventions	Rationales
Assess pain and proceed with conventional management of ischemic myocardial chest pain per institutional protocol.	Thrombolytic therapy does not preclude basic management aimed at decreasing pain, increasing myocardial oxygen supply and decreasing myocardial oxygen demand.
Determine the precise onset of symptoms that prompted medical care.	Maximizing the benefits of thrombolytic therapy requires early identification of the symptoms of AMI. The greatest benefit is obtained if initiated within 6 hr from onset of symptoms, as that is the time it takes for the affected portion of myocardial tissue to become necrotic.
	Note: Often patients will have episodes of waxing and waning chest pain that comes and goes or is relieved by rest or nitroglycerin. The window of opportunity before necrosis occurs begins when the pain becomes continuous and unrelenting, causing the patient to seek help.
Evaluate 12-lead ECG for characteristic changes of AMI.	

Nursing Interventions	**Rationales**
Evaluate cardiac enzymes. Treatment should not be delayed while awaiting the results of cardiac enzyme tests to confirm the diagnosis of AMI.	Serial enzyme evaluation is used as a method of supporting the initial diagnosis and monitoring the outcome following thrombolytic therapy. When reperfusion has occurred, the time to peak elevation of enzyme levels is approximately 12 hr after symptom onset. In contrast, the general time course to peak elevation in patients who do not reperfuse is approximately 24 hr.
Evaluate for contraindications to thrombolytic therapy. Refer to Table 3.1.	Thrombolytic therapy will not only dissolve an occlusive coronary thrombus, it will also lyse protective hemostatic clots throughout the vasculature. Careful assessment of these contraindications will avoid the development of potentially life-threatening hemorrhagic complications related to this therapy such as intracranial hemorrhage and internal bleeding. The risks of thrombolytic therapy should be weighed against the anticipated benefits.
Initiate institutional thrombolytic protocol. Do not waste significant amounts of time before giving the thrombolytic agent in order to obtain lab specimens or start IV lines. Time is critical. Clear explanations will help reduce anxiety	Prompt initiation of thrombolytic therapy is greatly enhanced by a written protocol on a "clot box" that contains all the necessary supplies and equipment.

Nursing Interventions	Rationales
Before initiating thrombolytic therapy: 1. Explain to patient/family the purpose of the therapy and that some minor bleeding may occur. 2. Draw appropriate lab specimens [chemistry panel, complete blood count (CBC), prothrombin/partial thromboplastin times (PT/PTT) fibrin split products, and cardiac enzymes]. 3. Determine baseline vital signs, neurological status, and pain level. 4. Establish at least two intravenous (IV) lines.	
Follow appropriate guidelines for the reconstitution, dosage, and administration of the specific thrombolytic agent.	
ACTIVASE (ALTEPLASE, RECOMBINANT) **Reconstitution** Aseptically add the appropriate volume of the accompanying sterile water for injection, USP, to the vial of Activase lyophilized powder.	It is important that Activase be reconstituted only with sterile water for injection, USP, without preservatives. Use of solutions containing preservatives (e.g., bacteriostatic water for injection, USP) during reconstitution may cause clouding of the Activase solution.
Direct the stream of sterile water directly into the cake of lyophilized powder using a large-bore needle (e.g., 18 gauge).	This action will facilitate the dissolution of the lyophilized powder into solution.
Follow package instructions for use of transfer device if using 100-mg vial of Activase.	
Complete the reconstitution process by gently rolling or inverting the vial of Activase. DO NOT SHAKE.	Gently rolling or inverting the vial of Activase will facilitate the complete dissolution of Activase into solution.

Nursing Interventions

Allow the reconstituted vial of Activase to stand undisturbed for a few minutes before further dilution and/or administration.

Examine the reconstituted solution of Activase before further dilution and/or administration.

Administer reconstituted Activase within 8 hr.

Dilution
Dilute the reconstituted solution (1 mg/mL) further to yield concentrations as low as 0.5 mg/mL where appropriate. Use normal saline or 5% dextrose in water (D_5W) for the diluent.

Do not add other medications to the Activase solution.

Use caution when purging IV tubing so as not to waste any drug.

Do not use buretrol or in-line filters.

Rationales

During reconstitution, some foaming may occur. Allowing the vial to sit undisturbed will promote dissipation of any bubbles into solution.

Reconstitution of the vial of Activase will result in a clear to pale yellow solution. Close examination of the vial will permit prompt recognition of any discoloration or cloudiness, which may indicate contamination or the presence of particulate matter.

This reconstituted solution of Activase (1 mg/mL) may be used for direct IV administration or it may be further diluted. Activase should not be reconstituted until just prior to its use (due to risk of bacterial growth) any unused portion should be discarded within 8 hr.

The infusion rate of a drug may be monitored and controlled more accurately when there is a larger volume of fluid to administer over time. Sterile water should not be used for further dilution. Further dilution of Activase with sterile water will result in a hypotonic solution and may cause the protein to precipitate.

Compatibility testing is not yet complete.

It is imperative that the patient receive the full "therapeutic dose."

It has been demonstrated that some filters can decrease the amount of Activase received by as much as 47%.

Nursing Interventions

Dosage/Administration
Administer the recommended dosage of Activase, 100 mg over 3 hr. [For a smaller patient (<65 kg), a dose of 1.25 mg/kg over 3 hr may be used.]

Administer Activase using the following recommended dosage regimen: lytic dose, 60 mg over the first hour, with 10% of the first hour's dose (6–10 mg) given as an IV push over 1–2 min.

Note: Reduce the rate of the activase infusion to the appropriate maintenance dose at the end of the first hour.

Administer maintenance dose—20 mg over the second hour followed by 20 mg over the third hour.

Flush the entire IV system with 25–30 mL of normal saline following the end of the Activase infusion. The fluid should be injected into the empty IV bag/bottle and infused at the final dosage rate.

Rationales

Studies evaluating Activase have shown that at a dose of 100 mg over 3 hr, coronary artery patency is achieved in approximately 71% of patients experiencing complete thrombotic occlusion of the infarct-related artery. Similar patency rates are being reported in studies using 100 mg Activase over 90 min with no increase in bleeding risk.

Dose-response studies with Activase have demonstrated that a lytic dose (approximately 60% of the total Activase dose) given over the first hour achieves rapid recanalization of the infarct-related artery. The 6–10-mg bolus dose is administered to bring circulating blood levels to a therapeutic range promptly. Begin the Activase drip immediately after the bolus, as it has an extremely short half-life of 5–6 min.

Following the 1-hr lytic infusion, the remainder of the Activase dose is delivered at a lower rate as a "maintenance" infusion. The goal is to maintain coronary artery patency and prevent rethrombosis.

To ensure the full dose of Activase has been delivered, the entire IV delivery system is flushed with additional fluid.

Nursing Interventions	Rationales

Readministration

Administer a follow-up dose per physician order taking the following into consideration:

1. amount of time elapsed since end of last Activase dose
2. patient/catheterization laboratory location and timing

If reocclusion occurs during Activase therapy, increase maintenance dose to 25 mg/hr per physician order and assist with arrangements for urgent cardiac catheterization and possible percutaneous transluminal coronary angioplasty (PTCA).

If reocclusion occurs within 6 hr of Activase, give 50–60 mg over 1 hr per physician order while assisting with arrangements for urgent cardiac catheterization.

If reocclusion occurs after more than 6 hr, it may be safe to give a full 100-mg dose while assisting with arrangements for urgent cardiac catheterization.

If reocclusion occurs while in a hospital with catheterization laboratory facilities, assist with the arrangement of immediate catheterization if possible. If delayed 30 min, start Activase as prescribed.

For visible filling defect, assist physician with administration of intracoronary Activase, 30 mg/15 min and additional 20 mg/10 min if necessary. Allow 15–20 min to detect the angiographic effects.

Reocclusion/reinfarction may occur after thrombolytic therapy in approximately 15% of cases. This is primarily due to the presence of high-grade stenosis.

Table 3.1 • Contraindications to Thrombolytic Therapy

Absolute Contraindication

Active internal bleeding (e.g., active peptic ulcer disease)

Severe uncontrolled hypertension

A known bleeding diathesis (e.g., thrombocytopenia, hemophilia)

Recent (within 2 months) intracranial or intraspinal surgery or trauma

Any history of cerebrovascular accident, intracranial neoplasm, arteriovenous malformation, or aneurysm

Receiving Eminase or streptokinase within the past 6 months (not applicable to Activase)

Relative Contraindications

Recent major surgery (within 10 days)

Cerebrovascular disease

Recent gastrointestinal or genitourinary bleeding (within 10 days)

Recent trauma (within 10 days)

Hypertension: systolic BP $\geq$ 180 mmHg and/or diastolic BP $\geq$ 110 mmHg

High likelihood of left-sided heart thrombus

Acute pericarditis

Subacute bacterial endocarditis

Significant liver dysfunction

Pregnancy

Diabetic hemorrhagic retinopathy

Septic thrombophlebitis

Advanced age (over 75 years)

Current use of oral anticoagulants

Any other condition in which bleeding constitutes a significant hazard or would be particularly difficult to manage because of its location

See full prescribing information of each of the agents for a complete list of contraindications and warnings to thrombolytic therapy.

Nursing Interventions	Rationales
STREPTASE (STREPTOKINASE) **Reconstitution.** Slowly add 5 mL sodium chloride, USP, or dextrose (5%), USP, to the streptokinase vial, directing the diluent at the side of the vacuum-packed vial rather than into the drug powder. Roll and tilt the vial gently to reconstitute. *Avoid shaking.* (Shaking may cause foaming.)	The protein nature and lyophilized form of streptokinase require careful reconstitution and dilution. Slight flocculation (described as thin translucent fibers) of reconstituted streptokinase may occur occasionally but do not interfere with the safe use of the solution.

Nursing Interventions	Rationales
Dilution Withdraw the entire reconstituted contents of the vial; slowly and carefully dilute further to a total volume of 45 mL. Avoid shaking and agitation of dilution.	If necessary, total volume may be increased to a maximum of 500 mL. To facilitate setting the infusion pump rate, a total volume of 45mL or a multiple thereof is recommended.
Visually inspect parenteral drug products for particulate matter and discoloration prior to administration.	The albumin (human) may impart a slightly yellow color to the solution.
Reconstitute immediately before use.	Streptokinase contains no preservatives; the solution may be used for direct IV administration within 8 hr following reconstitution if stored at 2–8 °C (36–46 °F).
Filter the reconstituted solution through a 0.8-μm or larger pore size filter.	
Do not add other medication to the container of streptokinase.	
Dosage/Administration. Administer the recommended dose of 1.5 million IU (45 mL) infused within 60 min (no weight adjusting).	

EMINASE (ANTISTREPLASE) **Reconstitution** Withdraw 5 mL of sterile water for injection, USP, using a 5- or 10-mL syringe.	
Inject the water slowly into the vial by directing the flow against the side of the vial.	
Gently roll the vial, mixing the powder and fluid. DO NOT SHAKE.	Gentle rolling of the vial will minimize foaming.
Inspect visually for particulate material or discoloration.	The material should be colorless to pale yellow and transparent.
Withdraw the entire contents of the vial (30 units) into the 5- or 10-mL syringe.	

Nursing Interventions	**Rationales**
Dilution Do not dilute further before administration.	
Do not add other medications to the vial or syringe containing Eminase	Compatibility studies are not yet complete.
Administration Administer the recommended dose of 30 units of Eminase (no weight adjusting).	
Begin administration as quickly as possible but not later than 30 min after reconstruction.	Eminase must be used within 30 min of being reconstituted or it begins to lose efficacy.
Administer by direct IV injection into the IV cannula, IV port, or stopcock closest to the patient.	
Inject Eminase slowly over 2–5 min. If IV fluids are being run, stop the flow of the main IV during the injection with Eminase.	
Flush the IV line with D_5W or normal saline (NS) after completing the injection with Eminase.	This is done to remove any remaining Eminase.
Administer acetylsalicylic acid (ASA) and heparin as ordered following administration of thrombolytic agent.	This provides sustained anticoagulant effect to minimize or prevent reocclusion. Heparin is particularly crucial in enhancing the patency rate of Activase because of its short half-life.
Evaluate for the occurrence of clinical markers of reperfusion, which usually occurs in 30–60 min:	

Nursing Interventions	Rationales
1. relief of chest pain	Nonthrombolytic pain relief typically occurs gradually over 6–8 hr and results from completed necrosis and/or narcotic analgesia and use of nitrates. In contrast, relief of chest pain associated with thrombolytic-induced reperfusion is usually rapid or abrupt in onset. The sudden or progressive relief usually occurs within 30 min of the first noted improvement in pain.
2. resolution of ST-segment elevation	The lead that demonstrated the greatest ST-segment elevation should be continuously monitored. Any sudden change in ST-segment elevation or other markers of reperfusion require an immediate 12-lead ECG. Resolution of ST-segment elevation occurs more rapidly and abruptly than that associated with a completed infarct.
3. development of dysrhythmias	The dysrhythmias most often observed include accelerated idioventricular rhythm, ventricular tachycardia, premature ventricular contractions, sinus bradycardia, and varying degrees of heart block.
Prepare patient for coronary catheterization to evaluate reperfusion.	The only way to definitely assess whether reperfusion has occurred is to perform coronary angiography, which allows direct visualization of the affected artery. However, PTCA has inherent risks and is not routinely recommended in the urgent phase. The nurse must rely on clinical markers of reperfusion. The greater the number of markers documented, the greater the predictive value. If one marker occurs, the nurse should continue to assess for the others.

NURSING DIAGNOSIS: HIGH RISK FOR FLUID VOLUME DEFICIT

Risk Factors
• Blood loss from dissolution of protective hemostatic clots

Patient Outcomes
Patient will exhibit stable blood pressure and pulse and minimal bleeding from puncture and other sites.

Nursing Interventions	Rationales
Assess the following: 1. all puncture sites and gingiva for evidence of bleeding 2. vital signs for evidence of hemodynamic instability 3. blood in stool, emesis, sputum, and urine for frank or occult blood 4. fibrinogen levels and PT/PTT levels (adjusting heparin to maintain PTT at 1.5–2 times control) 5. laboratory data for evidence of acute blood loss (Hgb, Hct). 6. postcardiac catheterization patients for evidence of muscle weakness, low back pain, and interruption of blood flow to lower extremities, indicating possible retroperitoneal bleeding	Bleeding may occur any place in the body where a protective clot has been dissolved.
Implement the following strategies to prevent excessive bleeding: 1. establish IV lines prior to initiating therapy. 2. draw laboratory specimens off of indwelling IV lines or capped IV line.	Inability to form hemostatic clots during the therapy may cause bleeding at puncture sites.

Nursing Interventions

3. avoid the following during therapy:
   - Insertion of invasive lines (preferable to wait 30 min after completion of the thrombolytic agent)
   - arterial punctures for arterial blood gases (ABGs)
   - intramuscular (IM) injections
   - discontinuing any arterial/ venous lines during thrombolytic therapy
   - IV blood sampling via puncture
   - excessive handling of patient during therapy
   - Automatic blood pressure cuffs
   - insertion of urinary catheter
   - vigorous tooth brushing
4. Use electric razor for the first 24 hr.
5. Place bleeding precautions sign at bedside.
6. Recommend prophylactic anti-ulcer therapy.

Rationales

During thrombolytic therapy bleeding may occur after even minimal trauma.

Nursing Interventions

Manage bleeding in the following manner:

1. Apply direct pressure to all arterial and venous puncture sites for a minimum of 30 min or until hemostasis is achieved.
2. Cover all venous and arterial access sites with a sterile, firm, pressure-type dressing.
3. Report any signs/symptoms of bleeding or hemodynamic instability to physician.
4. Discontinue the thrombolytic agent and heparin infusions in the presence of significant blood loss and/or hemodynamic compromise.
5. Initiate emergency therapy for significant fluid volume deficit per institutional protocol (e.g., Trendelenburg position, volume replacement, or blood product replacement).

Rationales

Superficial bleeding can be successfully managed by direct pressure. Surface or internal bleeding that results in fluid volume deficit or hemodynamic compromise requires emergency action and referral for definitive medical intervention. Due to the short half-life of Activase (5 min) and a clearance time of approximately 30 min, discontinuation of infusion will prevent further compromise of the patient's coagulation system. The anticoagulant effect of heparin will also contribute to bleeding, necessitating its discontinuation. The streptokinase agents have a sustained lytic state of 24–48 hr, which may present additional risks.

NURSING DIAGNOSIS: HIGH RISK FOR ALTERED TISSUE PERFUSION—CEREBRAL

Risk Factors
• Lysis of hemostatic clots in cerebral vasculature

Patient Outcomes
Patient will
• experience no neurological changes that would reflect an intracranial hemorrhage as a result of thrombolytic therapy.
• respond to early recognition and interventions to limit further alteration of symptoms of cerebral tissue perfusion.

Nursing Interventions	Rationales
Carefully screen for risks prior to initiating therapy. (Refer to Table 3.1.)	Patients who have a known or suspected history of cerebrovascular disorders are at increased risk for developing intracranial hemorrhage. The incidence of intracranial hemorrhage is very low (0.5%) when patients are properly screened.
Frequently assess for presence of headache, changes in mental status, neurological changes, and changes in vital signs for 24–48 hr following thrombolytic therapy.	These symptoms may be indicative of increased intracranial pressure due to intracranial bleeding.
Report any change in neurological status from baseline to physician immediately.	
Discontinue thrombolytic agent and heparin infusions if symptoms of increased intracranial pressure occur.	
Initiate emergency interventions to support vital physiological functions per institutional protocol.	

NURSING DIAGNOSIS: HIGH RISK FOR DECREASED CARDIAC OUTPUT

Risk Factors
- Reperfusion dysrhythmias

Patient Outcomes
Patient will
- maintain normal cardiac output as evidenced by a stable blood pressure and level of consciousness in spite of reperfusion dysrhythmias.
- respond to interventions for dysrhythmias and alterations in cardiac output.

Nursing Interventions	Rationales
Continuously monitor the ECG for dysrhythmias.	Reestablishment of blood flow to ischemic myocardium may be accompanied by dysrhythmias (PVCs, ventricular tachycardia, accelerated idioventricular rhythm, marked sinus bradycardia, or AV blocks).
Assess hemodynamic response to dysrhythmias.	Characteristically, "reperfusion" dysrhythmias are self-limiting or nonsustained, and aggressive antidysrhythmic therapy may not be necessary. However, the potential for decreased cardiac output does exist.
Provide early definitive management of sustained dysrhythmias per institutional protocol.	Dysrhythmias associated with reperfusion should be managed in the same way as any rhythm disturbance occurring during an AMI.
Keep antidysrhythmic therapy at bedside.	
Have defibrillator available.	
Notify physician of significant dysrhythmias.	

NURSING DIAGNOSIS: HIGH RISK FOR ALTERED TISSUE PERFUSION—MYOCARDIAL

Risk Factors
- Reocclusion/reinfarction of coronary artery

Patient Outcomes
Patient will
- remain free of chest pain and associated symptoms of recurrent myocardial ischemia.
- respond to interventions for coronary reocclusion/reinfarction.

Nursing Interventions	Rationales
Assess for the return of symptoms indicating myocardial ischemia. Reocclusion, rethrombosis of the infarct-related artery, may occur after successful thrombolysis.	Reocclusion occurs in approximately 12–15% of cases, usually within the first 24 hr. Signs and symptoms of reocclusion are exactly the same as symptoms of the original coronary occlusion.
Maintain the following therapies in order to prevent reocclusion/reinfarction: 1. Ensure that the thrombolytic agent is delivered at the appropriate dose and rate. 2. Monitor PT/PTT values in order to maintain a therapeutic range (1½–2× normal). 3. Administer ASA as ordered.	A combination of a thrombolytic agent, heparin, and ASA will achieve and help maintain a patent coronary artery.
Obtain a 12-lead ECG and compare with baseline for characteristic changes of ST-T waves and dysrhythmias indicating myocardial ischemia/reinfarction.	
Manage reocclusion/reinfarction by 1. immediately notifying physician of the return of any signs and symptoms associated with myocardial ischemia 2. administering appropriate pharmacological therapy for pain management and dysrhythmia control according to institutional protocol 3. preparing for possible emergency cardiac catheterization, repeat thrombolytic therapy, PTCA, and coronary artery bypass grafting (CABG).	Reocclusion/reinfarction represents a medical emergency similar to that caused by the initial MI. Patients should be managed appropriately under these conditions. Further therapy is directed at salvaging jeopardized myocardium and determining underlying pathology.

NURSING DIAGNOSIS: KNOWLEDGE DEFICIT (PATIENT/ SIGNIFICANT OTHER)

Related To lack of exposure to information about thrombolytic therapy

Defining Characteristics

Verbalizations that indicate inadequate understanding
Misinterpretation or misconceptions about thrombolytic therapy
Inadequate reporting of recurrent ischemic symptoms

Patient Outcomes

Patient will verbalize knowledge regarding
- the benefits and risks of thrombolytic therapy
- recognition and prompt reporting of recurrent ischemic symptoms

Nursing Interventions	Rationales
Prior to therapy, describe the following to patient/family: 1. Thrombolytics are medications that dissolve the blood clot in your coronary artery that is causing your heart attack. 2. The goal of this medicine is to limit the size of your heart attack.	Appropriate patient/family education can substantially reduce the anxiety and knowledge deficit associated with AMI and therapeutic intervention.
3. As a result of this therapy, you may experience some bruising and bleeding. Please help us monitor this.	Alerting the patient/family to the anticipated surface bleeding and bruising can dramatically reduce anxiety and promote optimal patient care.
4. During and following therapy, you will be closely observed for heart rhythm disturbances and evidence of bleeding. 5. During and following therapy, it is important to promptly notify the nurse of pain relief or any new onset of pain.	
Provide simple and concise answers to patient and/or family regarding therapy and patient's progress.	

DISCHARGE PLANNING/CONTINUITY OF CARE

- Instruct patient and family in the signs and symptoms of myocardial ischemia. The patient who cannot identify AMI symptoms and/or denies their presence often has the greatest delay in treatment.

- Emphasize that the primary goal is early treatment of recurrent AMI symptoms. Any unnecessary delay of time results in loss of cardiac muscle.
- Review mechanisms for obtaining medical care within their community. Emphasize the value of using the 911 rescue services if they are available.

REFERENCES

Anderson, J. L. (1990). Current approach to administering thrombolytic agent in acute MI: Approved protocols for use of three thrombolytic agents. *Journal of Critical Illness, 5*(1), 77–84.

Genentech. (1992). Activase (Alteplase, recombinant). 460 Point San Bruno Boulevard, South San Francisco, CA (drug prescribing information).

Hoechst-Roussel Pharmaceuticals. (l992). Streptase (streptokinase). Somerville, NJ (drug prescribing information)

Saul, L. (Ed.). (1991). *Activase therapy in AMI and acute massive pulmonary embolism: Nursing care guidelines.* American Association of Critical-Care Nurses Monograph. California: Gardiner-Caldwell Syner Med.

Smith Kline Beecham. (1990). Eminase (Anistreplase). Bristol, TN (drug prescribing information).

▼

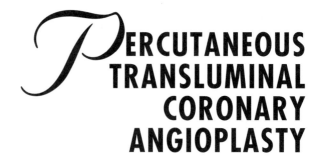

$\mathcal{P}$ERCUTANEOUS TRANSLUMINAL CORONARY ANGIOPLASTY

Lori A. Hislop, RN, BSN, CCRN

Percutaneous transluminal coronary angioplasty (PTCA) is an interventional method of opening a stenotic or occluded coronary artery. It has become a common treatment for coronary artery disease (CAD), the progressive obstruction of blood flow through one or more of the coronary arteries. This obstruction leads to deprivation of blood supply and therefore oxygen to the myocardium. Through the use of balloon-tipped catheters, the PTCA technique opens the coronary vessel, increasing myocardial oxygen supply.

Advances in balloon catheter technology and the introduction of rotational atherectomy, shaving atherectomy, lasers, and stents have expanded PTCA use in multivessel coronary disease. In addition, angioplasty of saphenous vein bypass grafts and internal mammary bypass grafts may be approached using this mechanism. The PTCA technique may also be utilized in the treatment of total coronary occlusions and in the setting of acute myocardial infarction (AMI). This technique has added a dimension to the treatment of coronary artery disease which was previously limited to surgical or medical approaches (Table 4.1).

ETIOLOGIES

Coronary artery disease
- Risk factors include smoking, male gender, advancing age, family history of CAD, obesity, diabetes mellitus, sedentary lifestyle, hypertension, hypercholesterolemia, and hypertriglyceridemia.
- Restenosis of a previous angioplasty site: a healing process involving deposition of smooth-muscle cells and fibroblasts at an angioplasty site. When this reparative process is excessive, it may encroach on the lumen of the coronary artery.
- Anastomotic site narrowing in coronary artery bypass graft (CABG)
- Progression of CAD in bypass graft (vein graft or internal mammary artery) or native coronary artery

Table 4.1 • Interventional Therapies in PTCA

Balloon angioplasty	Inflation of a balloon-tipped catheter in a coronary artery stenosis (plaque). This opens the lumen and restores blood flow to the distal myocardium.
Atherectomy	A high-speed diamond-tipped (rotational atherectomy) or shaving device (directional atherectomy) which removes plaque from the coronary artery. A shaving atherectomy removes plaque by way of a collection chamber within the catheter. Rotational atherectomy pulverizes the plaque into particles less than the size of the red blood cell and therefore may pass through the circulation. The action of the rotating burr may also hemolyze red blood cells. This may result in temporary hematuria as the cells are filtered out through the kidneys. Additionally, blood samples obtained immediately following rotational atherectomy may be hemolyzed. These samples should not be re-drawn as they will likely demonstrate evidence of hemolysis for several hours following the procedure. Atherectomy may be useful in treating heavily calcified lesions, total and subtotal occlusions, and long lesions.
Laser	A special type of light wave which can be controlled to carry energy in the form of heat. The laser waves are confined in an angioplasty catheter with the tip of the catheter being made of metal that heats when the laser is turned on. The laser catheter tip is placed across the lesion/blockage, the laser is turned on, and the subsequent heat production vaporizes the obstruction. Laser trials are being conducted in native coronary arteries as well as bypass grafts.
Stent	A stainless steel wire coil that acts as scaffolding device to give support to the artery and maintain patency. The stent is deployed to the site using a balloon angioplasty catheter. Stent(s) may be placed within native coronary arteries, saphenous vein bypass grafts, and internal mammary artery bypasses. The stent is currently undergoing investigational studies and its use is limited to those testing centers.

▼

CLINICAL MANIFESTATIONS

Decreased activity tolerance
- The patient describes a pattern of increasing fatigue and decreased ability to perform activities of daily living.

Angina pectoris (secondary to myocardial ischemia)
- Angina occurs when myocardial oxygen demand exceeds the arterial blood supply.
- The usual onset of angina is exertional in nature and is promptly relieved with rest and/or the use of sublingual nitroglycerin.
- The initial onset of angina is gradual and usually occurs over a 6–12-month period.
- Angina is often worsened when exertion follows a meal.
- Cold air or exposure to a sudden brisk wind may precipitate angina.
- The discomfort of anginal pain is highly variable but is commonly described as
  - a vague "bothersome" ache in the chest region
  - pain that may rapidly become severe
  - intense crushing sensation in precordial region
  - radiating pain to left shoulder and down left arm.
  - radiating pain to the back
  - radiating pain into throat, jaws, teeth, or right arm
  - possibly associated with abdominal pain, nausea, vomiting, bloating, and/or belching
  - possibly associated with shortness of breath, palpitations, and/or diaphoresis.

CLINICAL/DIAGNOSTIC FINDINGS

Noninvasive studies
- History and physical assessment
  - S_2 heart sound often becomes more parodoxic during episodes of myocardial ischemia due to prolonged left ventricular ejection.
  - S_4 heart sound is common and may be explained by ventricular filling, tensing of atrioventricular valve structures, and finally atrial muscle contraction produced in the presence of myocardial ischemia.
  - Occasionally a mid or late systolic apical murmur may be auscultated. This is related to papillary muscle dysfunction as a consequence of myocardial ischemia.
  - Heart sounds may become more distant during episode of chest pain related to myocardial ischemia.
  - Blood pressure usually elevates in the presence of myocardial ischemia.

- Hypertension may be found as a risk factor not previously diagnosed.
- Lung sounds may be clear; rales may suggest pulmonary congestion.
- Electrocardiogram (ECG)
  - evidence of previous myocardial injury (silent myocardial infarction)
  - evidence of ischemia (ST- and T-wave changes)
  - abnormalities that may include ST-segment depression, ST-segment elevation (hyperacute), T-wave inversion, decreased R-wave height, intraventricular or bundle branch conduction disturbances, dysrythmias (usually ventricular extrasystoles)
- Echocardiogram (ECHO)
  - Assess for wall motion abnormalities.
  - Left ventricular ejection fraction (LVEF) normally > 55%. Deterioration of ventricular performance may be noted, especially during episodes of ischemia.
  - Assess evidence for valvular insufficiency and/or evidence of valvular stenosis.
  - Rule out congenital heart disease.
- Chest x-Ray (CXR)
  - Identify cardiomegaly and pulmonary vascular congestion.
  - Assess the lung fields for alveolar and/or interstitial changes which may suggest preexisting pulmonary disease or dysfunction.
  - Identify aneurysm formation or calcification of the ascending aorta.

Laboratory Studies
- Lipid profile
  - Note elevation of cholesterol, triglygerides, and low-density lipoprotein (LDL).
  - High-density lipoprotein (HDL) may be normal or low.
- Complete blood count
  - Assess for undiagnosed anemia which may contribute to or explain the patient's angina.
- Electrolytes
  - Assess for hypokalemia which may provoke ventricular extrasystoles.
- Creatinine/blood urea nitrogen (BUN)
  - Assess for elevation of values that may indicate preexisting renal insufficiency which may require further investigation.
- Liver function studies
  - Assess for elevation of values which may point toward chronic liver congestion secondary to right-sided heart failure or may be consistent with primary liver dysfunction. The cause of abnormalities must be investigated as most primary medications are cleared through the liver.
- Stool for occult blood
  - A positive stool specimen should be investigated as to the source of occult loss. This is especially important if the patient needs to be placed on antiplatelet or anticoagulation therapy and/or if an anemia is also diagnosed.

Exercise stress testing

- Bruce protocol
  - Measures cardiac workload and vital sign response to exercise.
  - Uses treadmill exercise, continuous ECG, and physical assessment monitoring.
  - Diagnostic if clinical symptoms occur with associated ECG changes and/or changes in physical exam. Other diagnostic indicators include a decrease in exercise tolerance as compared to a previous study or based on the expected performance for that patient and his/her physical condition. Hypertensive response or exaggerated heart rate response to exercise may also be indicative of ischemia.
  - May be equivocal in the setting of preexisting ECG abnormalities such as atrial fibrillation or bundle branch block pattern.
- Thallium stress test
  - Uses treadmill exercise Bruce protocol (see above), continuous ECG, and physical assessment monitoring along with radioisotope scanning of the myocardium.
  - Positive thallium imaging will describe an area of reperfusion with rest as compared to exercise scan (during exercise ischemia limits the distribution of thallium to the affected area; this reperfuses at rest).
  - An area representing scar/fibrosis on the thallium image may represent preexisting infarcted tissue that does not perfuse at rest *or* exercise.
  - Thallium imaging is helpful to differentiate areas of ischemia in known or suspected multivessel CAD.
- First-pass rest and exercise (FPRE)
  - Measures the level of cardiac work and vital sign response to exercise.
  - Utilizes supine bicycle exercise along with continuous physical assessment.
  - Cardiolite isotope allows for nuclear imaging of the myocardium. In addition to perfusion, ejection fraction and wall motion may be assessed at both rest and exercise (with exercise-induced ischemia, wall motion abnormalities may be seen as well as a temporary decrease in ejection fraction as the left ventricular performance deteriorates).
  - This exam may be better tolerated in patients who are limited in their ability to walk on a treadmill.
  - FPRE is effective in evaluating multivessel coronary artery disease and will also establish the degree of loss of myocardial performance during exercise and the recovery at rest.
- Persantine/dobutamine thallium stress test
  - This is a "nonstress" stress test that utilizes continuous ECG and vital sign response to a pharmaceutical-induced stress on the heart.
  - This exam uses intravenous infusion of persantine or dobutamine to raise the blood pressure and heart rate and stresses the heart in a very controlled fashion.

- This exam is performed with the patient supine and because no physical exertion is required may be used for the patient who is physically unable to perform treadmill or supine bicycle exercise.
- Thallium imaging allows for assessment of myocardial perfusion at rest and exercise.

Invasive studies
- Cardiac catheterization
  - Injection of a contrast agent into the coronary system to evaluate coronary artery anatomy and identify critical stenoses; it measures right- and left-sided heart function and hemodynamic data.
  - Treatment options include angioplasty, surgery, or medical management.

NURSING DIAGNOSIS: HIGH RISK FOR DECREASED CARDIAC OUTPUT

Risk Factors
- Recent interventional procedure
- Myocardial ischemia

Patient Outcomes
- The patient will verbalize that he or she is free of chest pain or chest pain is controlled.
- The patency of the arterial lumen will be maintained through early intervention.
- The patient will
  - demonstrate hemodynamic stability as evidenced by stable vital signs, mentation unchanged from the baseline assessment, and urine output greater than 30 mL/hr.
  - be free of dysrhythmias.
  - respond to pharmacological therapies and be free of complications associated with their use.

Nursing Interventions	Rationales
Assess and document chest pain for site, intensity, and quality following the PTCA procedure.	Chest pain may be the first indication of acute closure of the coronary artery lumen, coronary spasm, or acute myocardial infarction. A "different" character of chest pain may represent a noncardiac source of pain that may require further evaluation (i.e., gastritis, esophagitis, gall bladder attack may produce similar but different types of pain).

Nursing Interventions	Rationales
Assess and monitor hemodynamic stability with continuous blood pressure and pulse monitoring (via arterial sheath to high-pressure line or noninvasive blood pressure cuff).	A change in vital signs may represent compromised left ventricular function in the setting of ischemia. A rapid deterioration in vital signs may occur and therefore continuous monitoring is essential.
Monitor telemetry continuously.	Coronary ischemia may be associated with a change in heart rhythm such as tachycardia, bradycardia, heart blocks, and ventricular ectopy.
Assess heart and breath sounds every hour for the first 4 hr following PTCA, then every 2–4 hr thereafter.	Changes from baseline assessment such as S_4 heart sound, paradoxical S_2 heart sound, rales, cough, dyspnea, or shortness of breath may be indicative of cardiac decompensation.
Monitor urine output hourly (if catheterized) or every 2–4 hr.	Decreased urine output (<30 mL/hr) may reflect poor renal perfusion.
Assess for jugular venous distention (JVD) with every vital sign check.	Distention of the jugular veins is reflective of increased right atrial pressure, a precursor to heart failure.
If chest pain occurs: 1. Apply oxygen at 2–4 L/min.	Supplemental oxygen may improve the oxygen supply to the tissues and end organs.
2. Administer nitroglycerin 1/150 grain sublingual. 3. Notify physician	Nitroglycerin acts as a vasodilator and relieves pain.
4. Administer morphine sulfate intravenously as prescribed.	Morphine is a vasodilator and will improve myocardial perfusion. It will also relieve pain and relax the patient, which reduces myocardial oxygen demand.
5. Administer calcium channel blocker (i.e., nifedipine 10 mg sublingual) as prescribed.	Calcium channel blockers will relieve coronary artery spasm if present.
6. Draw immediate creatine phosphokinase (CPK) isoenzyme; then draw 3 times every 8 hr or as prescribed.	Serial enzyme measurement assesses the degree of myocardial injury.

Nursing Interventions	**Rationales**
7. Perform immediate ECG.	Diagnostic changes indicative of ischemia (i.e., ST- or T-wave changes) may be identified.
8. Make the patient NPO.	There is a possibility of PTCA being repeated or emergency CABG being performed.
9. Place patient on bedrest.	Decreased activity will decrease the myocardial oxygen demand.
10. Stay with the patient. Provide calm, restful environment and provide reassurance.	This will allay patient anxiety. Keeping the environment quiet and calm will further decrease anxiety and therefore reduce myocardial oxygen demand.
Institute appropriate pharmacological therapy as prescribed. Monitor the response and assess for complications of use: 1. calcium channel blockers 2. beta blockers 3. nitroglycerin 4. heparin 5. inotropes 6. diuretics	See Table 4.2

NURSING DIAGNOSIS: HIGH RISK FOR ALTERED NORMAL CARDIAC ELECTRICAL CONDUCTION

Risk Factors
- Inadequate myocardial oxygen supply

Patient Outcomes
- The patient will be free of dysrhythmias or dysrhythmia is controlled.
- Cardiac output will remain adequate in the presence of rhythm disturbance as evidenced by stable vital signs, mentation unchanged from the baseline assessment, and urine output greater than 30 mL/hr.
- The patient will respond to pharmacological therapies and will be free of complications associated with their use.

Table 4.2 • Pharmacological Agents Commonly Used in PTCA

Calcium channel blocker	Inhibits calcium ion influx across the cardiac and smooth-muscle cells. Decreases myocardial contractility and oxygen demand. Dilates coronary arteries and arterioles.
Beta blocker	Reduces cardiac oxygen demand by blocking beta-catecholamine-induced increases in heart rate, blood pressure, and force of myocardial contraction.
Nitroglycerin	For acute anginal episode, reduces cardiac oxygen demand by decreasing left ventricular end-diastolic pressure. Decreases systemic vascular resistance (afterload). Dilates coronary vessels and also improves blood flow through collateral coronary vessels.
Heparin	Prevents clot formation at the PTCA site by accelerating the formation of an anti-thrombin III–thrombin complex. Inactivates thrombin and prevents the conversion of fibrinogen to fibrin.
Inotropes	For the treatment of failing left ventricle secondary to ischemia. Inotropic agents act to correct shock and restore hemodynamics. Inotropes increase cardiac output and improve blood flow to vital organs. Inotropes such as phenylephrine hydrochloride (Neo-Synephrine) may be used following rotational atherectomy to force embolized particles into the microcirculation. Though plaque is pulverized into particles less than the size of red blood cells, the distal embolization of "debris" may produce a temporary stunning of the left ventricle. Neo-Synephrine acts to restore blood pressure and force embolized particles into the microcirculation, thereby limiting the stunning effect.
Diuretics	For acute pulmonary edema secondary to ischemic left ventricle. Usual agent is a loop diuretic (furosemide, bumetanide, ethacrynic acid), which is the most potent and quick-acting agent. Loop diuretics inhibit sodium and chloride reabsorption at the proximal portion of the ascending loop of Henle.

Table 4.2 • Continued

Atropine	An anticholinergic which inhibits acetylcholine at a parasympathetice neuroeffector junction, this blocks the vagal effects on the sinoatrial node and enhances the conduction through the atrioventricular node, thereby accelerating heart rate. For the treatment of symptomatic bradycardia.
Lidocaine hydrochloride	Class Ib antiarrhythmic for the treatment of symptomatic or hemodynamically compromising ventricular extrasystoles. Acts to shorten the action potential.
Aspirin	Impedes clotting by blocking prostaglandin synthesis which prevents formation of the platelet-aggregating substance thromboxane A_2. Often administered daily in dose range 81–325 mg.
Advanced cardiac life support protocol	Follow protocol for dysrhythmia not responsive to first-line therapies.

Nursing Interventions	Rationales
Assess vital signs at the onset of dysrhythmia.	Checking the vital signs immediately upon onset is necessary to determine the effect upon cardiac output and to monitor the trend for signs of decompensation.
Assess level of consciousness, peripheral pulses, skin color, and temperature.	Comparing the level of consciousness to the baseline assessment determines if the cardiac output has affected mentation. The level of consciousness (LOC) may decrease, peripheral pulses will be diminished, skin may become pale or ashen, and skin temperature may become cool and/or clammy in the setting of decreased cardiac output.
Provide reassurance regarding the temporary nature of dysrhythmias following PTCA.	Reassurance may help allay anxiety and reduce oxygen demand.

Nursing Interventions	Rationales
Provide continuous telemetry monitoring for at least 24 hr following the PTCA.	If reperfusion dysrhythmias and/or acute closure of the vessel occurs, it usually happens within the first 24 hr following PTCA.
Follow routine monitored bed orders (institution policy) and emergency protocols such as advanced cardiac life support (ACLS).	Early institution of therapy for hemodynamically compromising rhythms will minimize complications associated with the rhythm.
Maintain temporary transvenous pacemaker (TVP) per institution policy.	Some PTCA and all rotational atherectomy procedures require the placement of TVP at the onset of the procedure. The high speed of the rotating burr and the potential for distal embolization in the distribution of the heart's conduction system may lead to temporary blocks in the heart rhythm.
Institute appropriate pharmacological therapy, assess response, and assess for complications associated with use: 1. atropine 2. lidocaine hydrochloride 3. ACLS protocol	See Table 4.2.

NURSING DIAGNOSIS: HIGH RISK FOR FLUID VOLUME EXCESS

Risk Factors
- Contrast dye load during PTCA
- Preexisting renal insufficiency
- Preexisting left ventricular dysfunction

Patient Outcomes
- Electrolytes, creatinine, and BUN will remain unchanged from the baseline assessment or will return to baseline at the time of discharge (2–4 days)
- Urine output of greater than 30 mL/hr or greater than 720 mL/24 hr will be maintained.
- Weight will remain unchanged from the baseline or return to baseline at the time of discharge.

Nursing Interventions	Rationales
Assess and report signs and symptoms of fluid overload (i.e., dyspnea, rales, peripheral edema, jugular venous distention) to the physician.	Contrast dye may precipitate acute tubular necrosis and transient renal failure leading to fluid volume excess and congestive heart failure.
Monitor laboratory values and report increased BUN, creatinine, and serum potassium.	Baseline values are necessary to follow the trends.
Alert the physician if the creatinine is greater than 1.3 mg/dL or if the patient is diabetic to consider intravenous hydration before the procedure.	Diabetes predisposes to renovascular disease and therefore a decreased ability to clear contrast agents.
Administer intravenous fluids as prescribed.	Hydration will assist in clearance of the contrast agent. In the setting of preexisting renal insufficiency, consideration may be given to hydration with Intravenous fluid 8–10 hr preprocedure.
Administer osmotic diuretics as prescribed.	Osmotic diuretics (i.e., mannitol 10%) may increase the osmotic pressure of glomerular filtration, inhibit tubular reabsorption of water and electrolytes, and elevate blood plasma osmolality resulting in enhanced flow of water into extracellular fluid. This increases circulating volume, promotes renal perfusion pressure, and as a consequence promotes diuresis. This promotes rapid clearance of the contrast agent and therefore limits the necrosing effect on the kidney tubule.
Encourage oral intake of fluids for the first 24 hr following the procedure.	Hydration is essential to assist in renal clearance of the contrast agent used.
Record hourly urine output if catheterized.	
Record 24 hr intake and output during the hospital course.	

Nursing Interventions	Rationales
Report urine outputs less than 30 mL/hr or less than 720 mL in 24 hr. Correlate with laboratory values.	A decrease in urine output may indicate decreased renal function. This may be related to the ability to clear the contrast or may be prerenal in origin (i.e., decreased perfusion from low cardiac output, dehydration).
Weigh daily and report weight gain of 2 lb in 24 hr or 5 lb in 48 hr to physician. Consider fluid restriction.	Rapid weight gain with renal insufficiency predisposes to congestive heart failure, especially if pre-existing left ventricular dysfunction is present.

NURSING DIAGNOSIS: HIGH RISK FOR INJURY

Risk Factors
Invasive arterial procedure may cause
- pseudoaneurysm formation
- hematoma
- thromboembolism
- infection

Patient Outcomes
- Peripheral pulses equivalent to the baseline assessment will be maintained.
- Vascular access site will remain clean, dry, and intact without erythema, drainage, or increased ecchymosis.
- Motion and sensation of the extremity used for access is unchanged from the baseline assessment.
- Body temperature will be less than 100 °F

Nursing Interventions	Rationales
Assess pulse, motion, and sensation at the entry site and distally with each vital sign check and prn.	A baseline assessment is used for comparison to each check. A sudden change may signal acute arterial occlusion and requires immediate intervention to avoid necrosis of tissue.
Monitor vital signs including temperature every 4 hr and prn. Report fever above 100 °F.	Fever may indicate infection.

Nursing Interventions	**Rationales**
Monitor hemoglobin, hematocrit, and white blood cell count.	A decrease in hemoglobin and/or hematocrit may indicate blood loss or anemia. Assess for source of loss. An elevated white blood cell count may signal an infection.
Mark hematoma size every hour and prn, and document changes in size. Use a skin marker to measure growth.	
Measure access site girth every hour and prn.	An increase may signal the development of a hematoma without obvious signs of external bleeding.
Auscultate for bruit over access site each shift.	A bruit may indicate pseudoaneurysm formation.
Perform ankle/brachial index prn (systolic ankle blood pressure divided by the systolic brachial pressure); normal, 0.95 or greater; mild to moderate arterial insufficiency, 0.50–0.70; and severe arterial insufficiency, <0.30.	The ankle/brachial index may give an objective value to lower extremity pulses and therefore may be valuable in assessing for changes in circulation to the extremity.
Report deterioration or absence of pulse in the extremity to the physician immediately.	Sudden loss of pulses in the extremity constitutes a medical emergency. Early institution of therapy will minimize complications.
Maintain the extremity in straight extended alignment for the duration of bedrest prescribed.	This avoids pressure at the access site and allows a platelet plug to form and seal the artery.
Following removal of access sheath, apply direct manual pressure for 20 min; then apply a dressing to the site for 8 hr.	Direct manual pressure assists in achieving hemostasis.
Following sheath removal and after hemostasis is obtained, apply a 10 lb sandbag over the site for 3 hr.	Because anticoagulation is used at the time of PTCA, the potential for late bleeding exists. Also, the presence of the sandbag "reminds" the patient not to move the affected extremity.

Nursing Interventions	Rationales
Post–sheath removal, maintain bedrest for 1. 8 hr—femoral approach 2. 3 hr—brachial approach	
Avoid elevation of the head of bed above 15°–30° for the first 8 hr following sheath removal (femoral approach).	Elevating the head of the bed may add additional pressure at the access site and may precipitate recurrence of bleeding. Skin folds over the abdomen and groin may obscure visualization of the site if the bed is elevated.

NURSING DIAGNOSIS: KNOWLEDGE DEFICIT

Related To complex treatment plan

Defining Characteristics
Verbalizations indicating inadequate understanding, misinterpretation of information, or misconception of desired health behavior
Lack of recall of information given
Inability to follow instructions

Patient Outcomes
The patient (and family) will
- verbalize routine PTCA procedures.
- verbalize understanding of investigational procedures (i.e., intracoronary stents, rotational atherectomy, or laser) that may be used during the procedure.
- verbalize knowledge of emergency CABG procedures.
- notify staff immediately of any symptom or problem.
- comply with postprocedure follow-up and care.

Nursing Interventions	Rationales
Assess the patient and family's knowledge of procedures.	Knowledge is assessed so appropriate content and teaching strategies can be planned.
Present information from a standardized teaching plan for PTCA procedures and document teaching done. See Table 4.3.	

Nursing Interventions	Rationales
Encourage questions and verbalization of concerns and fears. Ask open-ended questions and allow adequate time to discuss concerns.	
Instruct the patient and family in routine protocols for CABG standby for emergency procedure.	Although rarely needed, the patient and family must understand that complications requiring emergency open heart surgery are possible.
Explain the importance of reporting subjective symptoms (i.e., chest pain, pain at access site, shortness of breath) immediately. Emphasize that time is critical when dealing with complications.	The patient may fear further procedures or may deny symptoms.
Review investigational procedures and permits verbally and provide written information. Allow adequate time for reading and reviewing materials.	
Begin discharge teaching and planning. Include 1. risk factor modification 2. follow-up protocols and procedures 3. restenosis versus progression of disease	

▼

Table 4.3 • Teaching Plan for PTCA Procedures

Patient will be able to:

- Define risk factors for coronary artery disease (CAD).
- Assist in identifying his or her risk factors for CAD.
- Prioritize his or her risk factors and focus on lifestyle-modifying behaviors specific to these.
- Discuss the purpose of PTCA and the expected outcome. Emphasize that CAD is progressive and there is no cure, but progression can be minimized with risk factor modification.
- Verbalize the significance of chest pain:
  - May be expected during balloon inflations; however, it is expected to abate.
  - Chest pain may signal acute/abrupt closure of the artery.
  - Importance of informing staff if any chest pain occurs at any time.
- Describe the sequence of events expected during and following PTCA:
  - Review of angiogram.
  - Patient will be awake (or lightly sedated) for the procedure; use of local anesthetic at access site.
  - May be asked to cough or hold breath during the procedure.
  - Significance of chest pain during the procedure.
  - Return to a monitored area following procedure.
  - May eat after fully awake.
  - Use of intravenous medications.
  - Frequency of vital sign checks and assessment of peripheral pulse.
  - Manual pressure, sandbags, and clamps to access site following sheath removal.
- Discuss angina and define what causes angina pain.
- Discuss how nitroglycerin works to relieve angina and why it is important to take at the onset of pain.
- List current medications, reason for administration, and desired effect. Discuss possible side effects.
- Discuss the use of anticoagulation and/or antiplatelet medications. Recognize the importance of compliance with lab draws, dose schedule, and ongoing communications with the physician/nurse.
- Arrange for follow-up testing: frequent stress testing within the first year following angioplasty and at least yearly thereafter.
- Recognize that CAD is progressive and early identification of problems can impact on mortality and morbidity of the disease. Frequent visits with the physician and perhaps repeat cardiac catheterization may be necessary.
- Define restenosis. Discuss the risk, benefits, and possible complications of PTCA, including (but not limited to) bleeding, infection, stroke, heart attack, or acute closure of an artery, which may require emergency bypass surgery. Discuss the use of CABG in an emergency situation. Differentiate between acute closure and restenosis (chronic closure) of an artery.
- Verbalize feelings about PTCA and the possibility of CABG.

▼

DISCHARGE PLANNING/CONTINUITY OF CARE

- Review patient's pre-PTCA learning needs and assess current knowledge. Correct misconceptions and reinforce information.
- Include spouse, family members, and significant others in discharge teaching.
- Prepare a road map of medications, dosages, and dose schedule. Ensure that the patient is sent home with necessary prescriptions.
- Assess the need for community resources and provide with appropriate referrals.
- Encourage participation in cardiac rehabilitation. Secure prescription and directions for cardiac rehabilitation from the physician prior to discharge.
- Consult the dietitian to meet with the patient and spouse/significant other to review recommended dietary guidelines.
- Review the patient's risk factors list (identified on admission) and assess strategies to alter his or her risks for CAD. Ask the patient to verbalize one or two lifestyle modifications for each risk factor identified.
- Discuss warning signals and possible complications requiring immediate attention:
  - prolonged episode of chest pain (pain unrelieved by three sublingual nitroglycerin tablets/sprays in a 15-min period)
  - weight increase of 2 lb in 1 day or 5 lb in 2 days
  - acute episode of shortness of breath or a new onset of increasing exertional dyspnea
  - bleeding from access site
- Review mechanism to access emergency response system:
  - Dial 911 (or call ambulance/fire department based on local availability).
  - Encourage patients to keep physician's name and phone number with them at all times (i.e., wallet identification card).
  - Provide written schedule for follow-up appointments and stress testing at the time of discharge.

REFERENCES

Cequier, A., Bonan, R., Crepeau, J., Cote, G., De Guise, P., Joly, P., Lesperance, J., & Waters, D. (1988). Restenosis and progression of coronary atherosclerosis after coronary angioplasty. *Journal of the American College of Cardiology, 12*(1), 49–55.

Loan, T. (1986). Nursing interaction with patients undergoing coronary angioplasty. *Heart & Lung, 15*(4), 368–375.

Popma, J., & Dehmer, G. (1989). Care of the patient after coronary angioplasty. *Annals of Internal Medicine, 110*(7), 547–558.

Sipperly, M. E. (1989). Expanding role of coronary angioplasty: Current implications, limitations, and nursing considerations. *Heart & Lung, 18*(5), 507–513.

$\mathcal{C}$ONGESTIVE HEART FAILURE

Mary G. Schigoda, RN, MSN, CCRN

Congestive heart failure (CHF) is a clinical syndrome in which there is inadequate cardiac output (CO) to meet the metabolic demands of the body, resulting in poor perfusion to all organ systems. CHF results from any condition that reduces the heart's ability to pump. Physiologically, this results in diminished forward flow and pooling of blood behind the left and/or right ventricle(s).

ETIOLOGIES

- Primary muscle disease
  - cardiomyopathy, myocarditis
- Secondary myocardial dysfunction
  - coronary artery disease with ischemia/infarction, biochemical alterations (low calcium, magnesium)
- Congenital, rheumatic, or acquired valvular disease
  - aortic, mitral, pulmonic, or tricuspid insufficiency or stenosis
- Congenital anomalies
  - atrial or ventricular septal defect, patent ductus arteriosus, arteriovenous fistula
- Obstructive disorders
  - idiopathic hypertrophic subaortic stenosis, coarctation of the aorta, hypertension
- Restrictive disorders
  - cardiac tamponade, restrictive pericarditis
- Endocrine/metabolic disorders
  - thyrotoxicosis, anemia, fever, pregnancy, systemic infection, beriberi, Paget's disease

CLINICAL MANIFESTATIONS

Right-sided heart failure
- Jugular venous distention (JVD)

- Elevated central venous pressure (CVP) and right atrial pressure (RAP)
- Splenomegaly
- Hepatomegaly
- Hepatojugular reflex
- Abdominal distention
- Anorexia
- Nausea/vomiting
- Ascites
- Peripheral edema
- Weight gain

Left heart failure
- Breathlessness
- Orthopnea
- Dyspnea on exertion (DOE)
- Paroxysmal nocturnal dyspnea (PND)
- Nocturia
- Decreased urine output (UO)
- Diaphoresis
- Cough
- Crackles, wheezes, or pleural fluid
- Hemoptysis
- Cyanosis
- Cheyne-Stokes breathing
- Palpitations
- Tachycardia
- Dysrhythmias
- Elevated pulmonary capillary wedge pressure (PCWP) and left atrial pressure (LAP)
- Gallop rhythm (S_3)

CLINICAL/DIAGNOSTIC FINDINGS

Noninvasive tests
- Electrocardiography (ECG)
  - tachycardia
  - atrial and/or ventricular ectopy
  - atrial and/or ventricular enlargement
  - ischemia/infarction
- Echocardiography (ECHO)
  - dilatation of cardiac chambers
  - atrial, ventricular, septal hypertrophy
  - valvular insufficiency and/or stenosis
  - septal and left ventricular free wall motion abnormalities (akinesis, hypokinesis, paradoxical motion)
  - decreased left ventricular ejection fraction (LVEF) (norm: 55–70%)

- Chest x-ray (CXR)
  - cardiomegaly
  - pulmonary vascular congestion
  - alveolar or interstitial edema
  - pleural effusions
- Multigated blood pool imaging (MUGA) scan
  - wall motion abnormalities
  - decreased right ventricular ejection fraction (RVEF) and/or LVEF
- Electrolytes
  - Na low (dilutional or due to diuretics)
  - K high (due to renal insufficiency)
  - Cl low (dilutional or due to diuretics)
  - CO_2/HCO_3 low (metabolic acidosis due to impaired tissue perfusion), high (metabolic alkalosis due to diuretic therapy)
- Renal function tests (RFTs)
  - blood urea nitrogen (BUN) elevated
  - creatinine elevated
  - creatinine clearance low
  - urine specific gravity elevated
- Liver function tests (LFTs)
  - lactate dehydrogenase (LDH) elevated
  - serum glutamic oxaloacetic transaminase/pyruvic transaminase (SGOT/SGPT) elevated
  - total bilirubin elevated
  - prothrombin time prolonged
- Complete blood count (CBC)
- – WBC (leukocytosis)
  - RBC (polycythemia)
  - Hgb/Hct (anemia)
- Arterial blood gases (ABGs) acid-base balance
  - pH low (due to metabolic acidosis)
  - HCO_3 low (due to metabolic acidosis)
  - Pao_2 low (due to pulmonary congestion)
  - $Paco_2$ low (due to respiratory alkalosis), high (due to respiratory acidosis)

Invasive tests
- Right-sided heart catheterization
  - high pulmonary artery/capillary wedge pressure (PAP/PCWP) (due to hemodynamic dysfunction)
- Left-side heart catheterization
  - low LVEF and CO/cardiac index (CI), high left ventricular end diastolic pressure (LVEDP) (due to hemodynamic dysfunction)
  - aortic/mitral insufficiency or stenosis (due to valve dysfunction)
- Coronary angiography
  - coronary artery disease (CAD) induced ischemia resulting in decreased contractility

NURSING DIAGNOSIS: DECREASED CARDIAC OUTPUT

Related To diminished ventricular performance

Defining Characteristics
Abnormal ABGs
Abnormal CXR
Abnormal electrolytes
Abnormal heart sounds (S_3, S_4)
Angina
Cough
Crackles
Cyanosis; pallor of skin and mucous membranes
Decreased activity tolerance
Decreased peripheral pulses
Dyspnea
Dysrhythmias; other electrocardiographic changes
Edema (peripheral and pulmonary)
Ejection fraction < 40%
Fatigue
Jugular vein distention
Oliguria; anuria
Orthopnea
Paroxysmal nocturnal dyspnea
Shortness of breath
Syncope
Variations in blood pressure
Variations in hemodynamic parameters
Weakness
Weight gain

Other Possible Characteristics
Abdominal distention
Anorexia
Ascites
Change in mentation/level of consciousness
Diaphoresis
Anxiety/fear
Frothy sputum
Left parasternal lift
Palpitations
Restlessness

Patient Outcomes
Patient will
- demonstrate hemodynamic stability as evidenced by hemodynamic parameters within normal limits (WNL) (see Table 5.1)

- respond to appropriate pharmacological therapy and not experience complications from the administration of inotropic agents, vasodilators, or diuretics.
- demonstrate a reduction in anxiety or fear from diagnostic tests/ procedures.
- demonstrate a reduction in cardiac workload.
- maintain normal fluid and electrolyte balance.

Table 5.1 • Normal Hemodynamic Parameters

Hemodynamic Parameters	Normal Values
$CO = HR \times SV$	4–8 L/min
$CI = CO/BSA$	2.5–3.5 L/min/m^2
$SV = CO/HR$	55–100 mL/beat
$MAP = Systolic + 2(diastolic)/3$	70–105 mmHg
$SVR = (MAP - RAP)/CO \times 80$	800–1200 dyn/cm/s^{-5}
$PVR = (MPAP - PCWP)/CO \times 80$	60–100 dyn/cm/s^{-5}
RAP (mean)	0–7 mmHg
LAP (mean)	6–12 mmHg
PAP	15–25/8–15 mmHg
PCWP (mean)	6–12 mmHg
HR	60–100 bpm

Note: CO = cardiac output, HR = heart rate, SV = stroke volume, CI = cardiac index, BSA = body surface area, MAP = mean arterial pressure, SVR = systemic vascular resistance, RAP = right atrial pressure, PVR = pulmonary vascular resistance, MPAP = mean pulmonary artery pressure, PCWP = pulmonary capillary wedge pressure, LAP = left atrial pressure, PAP = pulmonary artery pressure, .

Nursing Interventions	Rationales
Monitor hemodynamic stability by assessing 1. mean arterial pressure (MAP)	Circulating volume needs to be sufficient to maintain systolic blood pressure at 80–90 mmHg, or no more than 30 mmHg below hypertensive patient's usual pressure. Decreased pressure may result in hypoperfusion of the myocardium resulting in ischemia and decreased contractility.

Nursing Interventions	**Rationales**
2. CO/CI	Cardiac output is a measurement of cardiac function influenced by preload, afterload, contractility, and heart rate. Cardiac index is a more specific determinant of CO as it considers body size.
3. right atrial pressure (RAP) or central venous pressure (CVP)	Elevation suggests volume overload and/or heart failure (in the absence of volume overload).
4. PAP	Elevation reflects pulmonary congestion, which may lead to right-sided heart failure.
5. PCWP	Elevation exceeding 16–18 mmHg reflects pulmonary congestion and left-sided heart failure.
6. heart rate and rhythm	Significant dysrhythmias may occur as a result of depressed myocardial contractility leading to ischemia and decreased coronary perfusion, electrolyte imbalances, catecholamines, and drug toxicity (e.g., digoxin).
7. heart sounds	The S_3 and S_4 (abnormal) heart sounds are associated with rapid filling of a noncompliant ventricle. They may be muffled in the presence of an acute infarct or pulmonary congestion.
8. breath sounds	Crackles, rhonchi, and wheezes may be due to fluid accumulation and bronchospasm resulting from the pulmonary hypertension and congestion that occur when the left ventricle fails.
9. body/skin temperature	Elevations in temperature increase myocardial oxygen consumption and may result in ischemia and further depression of myocardial contractility, decreasing CO. Cool, clammy skin may be due to peripheral vasoconstriction
10. UO	Decreased UO occurs as the body attempts to compensate for decreasing CO by the reabsoption of sodium/water.

Nursing Interventions	Rationales
11. JVD	Increased RAP impedes flow of venous blood from vena cava. Inadequate venous drainage is manifested by distended neck veins.
12. edema, ascites, hepatic congestation	Fluid shifts occur as a result of hypotension, decreased glomerular filtration, and capillary membrane changes in response to humoral changes associated with heart failure.
Administer appropriate diuretic(s) as prescribed (see Table 5.2)	Diuretic agents increase the elimination of sodium and water by the kidney, resulting in a decrease in vascular volume and left ventricular (LV) filling pressure (preload).
Assess response to diuretic therapy, monitoring for 1. decrease in orthopnea, DOE, PND, and peripheral edema	Decreasing circulating volume relieves pulmonary and systemic congestion resulting in improved hemodynamics and respiratory status.
2. increase in UO and decrease in weight, abdominal girth, JVD, pulmonary crackles, and S_3 gallop 3. decrease in PCWP and CVP/RAP	
If resistance to diuretic therapy occurs: 1. Administer combination of diuretics that have differing sites of action within the kidney.	Combination therapy will restore diuresis by altering sodium reabsorption throughout major portions of the nephron.
2. Administer higher doses of loop diuretics and/or combination therapy.	Drug delivery to site of action decreases as renal function decreases. Note: Thiazide diuretics are ineffective in patients with creatinine clearances below 30 mL/min, with the exception of metalozone, which can be used without hesitation.

Nursing Interventions	**Rationales**
3. Restore depleted protein stores, monitor colloid osmotic pressure (COP), with slow, cautious diuresis (1 kg/day in most patients; 1 lb/day in patients with ascites).	Diuresis is more difficult in patients with decreased albumin levels due to decreased COP. If diuresis is too aggressive, volume depletion may occur despite overt edema.
Monitor for/treat complications of diuretic therapy:	
1. Treat hypokalemia (lethargy, somnolence, weakness, muscle cramps, dysrhythmias) with oral/IV potassium supplement.	Increased potassium excretion occurs due to increased sodium and water delivery to the distal tubule.
2. Treat hypomagnesemia with oral/IV magnesium.	Hypomagnesemia often occurs with decreased potassium. It must be replenished prior to potassium replacement or potassium will remain low despite high doses of supplement.
3. Treat hyponatremia (lethargy, somnolence, weakness) by restricting fluids and temporarily stopping diuretic therapy.	Hyponatremia occurs due to an imbalance between water intake and renal diluting capacity.
4. Treat metabolic alkalosis by reducing diuretic dose.	Metabolic alkalosis may occur when hypokalemia is accompanied by contraction of extracellular fluid volume and absorption of bicarbonate.
5. Treat hyperuricemia (elevated serum uric acid levels) by discontinuing diuretics. (If patient requires diuretic therapy and is symptomatic, may try allopurinol.)	Hyperuricemia is seen with chronic administration of thiazide and loop diuretics but is seldom a problem requiring additional treatment.
6. Administer large IV doses of loop diuretics slowly (e.g., furosemide 40 mg/min and bumetanide 1 mg/min) and do not use concurrently with aminoglycoside antibiotics (e.g., gentamycin, tobramycin.	These actions may prevent ototoxicity associated with high doses of loop diuretics.
7. Monitor blood sugar levels for detection of carbohydrate intolerance.	Carbohydrate intolerance occurs in some patients receiving chronic thiazide diuretic therapy. It may pose problems for latent diabetics.

Nursing Interventions	Rationales
8. Monitor for bone marrow suppression, hyperlipidemia, and impotence with loop and thiazide diuretics. Gynecomastia may be seen with long-term, high-dose spironolactone therapy.	These are rare side effects but do not occur in a small percentage of those on diuretic therapy.
Administer appropriate vasodilators as prescribed (See Table 5.3).	Vasodilators decrease vasoconstriction, resulting in the reduction of preload and/or afterload. In patients with decreased contractility, reducing preload and afterload leads to increased stroke volume (SV) and CO.
Assess response to vasodilator therapy, monitoring for 1. decrease in MAP, RAP/CVP, and PCWP 2. decrease in systemic vascular resistance (SVR) and pulmonary vascular resistance (PVR) 3. increase in SV and CO 4. increase in exercise tolerance 5. decrease in dyspnea and pulmonary congestion	Vasodilation decreases preload and afterload, resulting in improved hemodynamics.
Monitor for/treat complications of vasodilator therapy: 1. Observe for headache, flushing, palpitations, and dizziness; treatment usually is not necessary. 2. Observe for nausea, vomiting, and exacerbation of angina. 3. Observe for signs/symptoms of drug-induced systemic lupus erythematosis. Discontinue hydralazine if symptoms occur. 4. Observe for signs/symptoms of thiocyanate toxicity (confusion, convulsions, metabolic acidosis, lethargy) in the patient on nitroprusside therapy.	These common side effects of nitrates and hydralazine are usually mild and transient. These side effects occur in 20–30% of patients on long-term hydralazine therapy. Lupus like symptoms can occur after prolonged hydralazine therapy with high doses (>400 mg/day). Infusion rates below 3 μg/kg/min for under 72 hr are normally not associated with toxicity. Thiocyanate levels above 10 mg/dL are considered toxic.

Nursing Interventions	Rationales
5. Monitor fluid volume status.	Vasodilation can decrease circulating blood volume, resulting in hypotension.
6. Treat hypotension with normal saline (NS) infusion.	Normal saline prevents fluid from shifting into the interstitial space, restoring blood volume and pressure.
7. Hold/taper diuretics for 24 hr.	Ensures adequate filling pressures.
8. Monitor for proteinuria and nephrotic syndrome; discontinue angiotension converting enzyme (ACE) inhibitors if renal effects occur.	Renal dysfunction may occur in patients on long-term ACE inhibitor therapy.
9. Treat hyperkalemia by decreasing dose or discontinuing ACE inhibitors and/or potassium-sparing diuretics.	Hyperkalemia may develop in patients concomitantly taking ACE inhibitors and potassium-sparing diuretics.
Administer appropriate inotropic agents (see Table 5.4).	Inotropic agents increase contractility, resulting in increased CO and decreased LVEDP
Assess response to inotropic therapy by monitoring for 1. enhanced UO and weight loss 2. increased blood pressure and CO 3. decreased PCWP and SVR/PVR	Increased contractility improves renal blood flow, resulting in enhanced urine production, weight loss, and overall improvement in hemodynamics.
Monitor for/treat complications of inotropic therapy: 1. Observe fors signs/symptoms of digitalis toxicity (nausea, vomiting, anorexia, malaise, headache, altered vision, and dysrhythmias), especially in patients with renal insufficiency. 2. Treat digitalis toxicity by discontinuing the drug, optimizing serum potassium levels, a temporary pacemaker, and digoxin antibody, if appropriate.	Digitalis is metabolized and excreted through the kidneys. Levels exceeding 2.0 mg/mL are generally considered toxic.

Nursing Interventions	**Rationales**
3. Decrease dopamine/dobutamine dose if palpitations, chest pain, and/or decrease in blood pressure and CO occur.	Pain, palpitations, and decreased blood pressure/CO may occur with higher dose dopamine/dobutamine therapy due to the increase in myocardial oxygen consumption.
4. Monitor platelet counts.	Thrombocytopenia occurs in approximately 4% of patients receiving amrinone therapy.
5. Monitor liver function tests.	Liver function abnormalities are seen occasionally in patients on long-term amrinone therapy.
Implement other interventions to reduce work of the heart:	
1. Assess for reduction in cardiac workload by monitoring • exercise/activity tolerance • hemodynamic parameters	A reduction in workload lessens myocardial oxygen consumption and minimizes fatigue.
2. Maintain accurate intake and output (I&O)	Decreasing UO may be indicative of compensation for decreasing CO.
3. Weigh daily on the same scale at same time in the same clothes.	Weight gain may reflect fluid retention indicative of worsening heart failure.
4. Explain all diagnostic tests and procedures to minimize anxiety and fear.	Anxiety/fear can precipitate stress response characterized by catecholamine release, resulting in increased myocardial oxygen consumption.
5. Explain need for fluid restriction.	Restricting fluid intake (oral and IV) reduces circulating blood volume.
6. Teach importance of low sodium diet.	Restricting sodium intake minimizes fluid retention.
7. Teach energy-conserving stategies.	Decreasing exercise/activity tolerance reflect decreasing CO.
8. Assist with mechanical fluid removal, such as hemofiltration, if response to pharmacological and other interventions is inadequate.	

NURSING DIAGNOSIS: IMPAIRED GAS EXCHANGE

Related To pulmonary vascular congestion

Defining Characteristics

Agitation
Bradypnea
Central cyanosis
Confusion
Decreased ability to concentrate
Decreased oxygen saturation
Depression
Dyspnea
Fatigue
Forgetfulness
Hypercapnea
Hypoxemia
Increased or decreased blood pressure
Increased or decreased CO/CI
Increased or decreased SRV
Irritation
Restlessness
Somnolence
Stupor
Tachypnea

Table 5.2 • Specific Mechanisms of Action of Diuretics Used to Treat CHF

Types of Diuretics	Mechanism of Action
Thiazide diuretics: metolazone, hydrochlorothiazide, chlorothiazide	Moderately potent diuretics which inhibit sodium reabsorption in the distal tubules and increase potassium excretion in the distal and collecting ducts.
Loop diuretics: ethacrynic acid, furosemide, bumetamide	Most potent diuretics currently available; act by inhibiting chloride transport in the thick ascending loop of Henle.
Potassium-sparing diuretics: spironolactone, amiloride, triamterene	Weak diuretics; spironolactone competively inhibits aldosterone and produces mild diuresis; amiloride and triamterene work independent of aldosterone to inhibit sodium transport in the distal convoluted tubules.

Table 5.3 • Specific Mechanisms of Action of Vasodilators Used to Treat CHF

Vasodilators	Mechanism of Action
Angiotensin converting enzyme (ACE) inhibitors: captopril, enalapril maleate, lisinopril	The ACE inhibitors decrease both preload and afterload by lowering production of angiotensin II, a potent vasoconstrictive peptide and by decreasing the degradation of bradykinin, an endogenous vasodilating substance. Reduction of angiotensin II results in decreased mean arterial, central venous, and left ventricular end-diastolic pressures and increased stroke volume (SV) and cardiac output (CO). Production of aldosterone (a sodium-retaining and potassium-wasting hormone) is decreased, reducing the volume expansion usually seen with other vasodilators. The ACE inhibitors also increase renal blood flow (RBF) and glomerular filtration rate (GFR), promoting diuresis and lowering diuretic requirements in most patients. Other effects include decreasing levels of circulating catecholamines, increasing prostaglandin production, and decreasing vasopressin secretion.
Nitrates: Isosorbide dinitrate, nitroglycerin	Nitrates are primarily venodilators but at higher doses also dilate arterial smooth muscle. Their major hemodynamic effect is to decrease preload, improving exercise tolerance, pulmonary congestion, and dyspnea.
Hydralazine	Hydralazine is a direct acting arterial vasodilator. Its major hemodynamic effects are decreasing systemic and pulmonary vascular resistance (SVR, PVR) and increasing SV and CO.
Nitroprusside	Nitroprusside is an intravenous agent that has balanced vasodilating effects on the arterial and venous systems. Major hemodynamic effects include decreasing SVR and PVR and increasing SV and CO.

▼

Table 5.4 • Specific Mechanisms of Action of Inotropic Agents Used to Treat CHF

Inotropic Agents	Mechanism of Action
Digitalis	The digitalis glycosides inhibit the sodium-potassium adenosinetriphosphatase (ATPase) pump, which results in increased transport of calcium into the cell. The major hemodynamic effect is to increase cardiac output (CO).
Dopamine	Dopamine is an endogenous catecholamine that increases myocardial contractility by directly stimulating beta receptors. It indirectly releases norepinephrine from nerve terminals. Its effects are dose dependent. Low doses (<2.0 μg/kg/min) selectively stimulate dopamine receptors, resulting in enhanced renal blood flow (RBF) and diuresis. Moderate doses (2.0–10.0 μg/kg/min) stimulate both dopamine and beta receptors, resulting in enhanced RBF, diuresis, and CO. High doses (>10.0 μg/kg/min) cause stimulation of alpha receptors. Increases in systemic vascular resistance (SVR) and blood pressure usually offset any improvement in RBF or CO and may actually worsen these parameters.
Dobutamine	Dobutamine is a $beta_1$ selective agent that directly stimulates beta receptors to increase contractility. The major hemodynamic effects include increased CO, decreased pulmonary capillary wedge pressure (PCWP), and increased RBF. The amount of change seen in RBF and PCWP is directly related to the amount of change in CO. Its action is not dose dependent. Intermittent or continuous therapy may be used.
Amrinone	Amrinone inhibits myocardial cellular phosphodiesterase and increases the availability of calcium in the myocardium. It also decreases SVR, although the exact mechanism by which this occurs is not known. Its major hemodynamic effects are decreased SVR and PCWP and increased CO and RBF.

▼

Table 5.5 • Normal Arterial Blood Gas Values

Value	Normal Ranges
pH	7.36–7.44
Paco$_2$	36–44 mmHg
Pao$_2$	95–100 mmHg
HCO$_3$	22–28 mmol/L

Note: pH = expression of the acid-base balance; Paco$_2$ = partial pressure of carbon dioxide; Pao$_2$ = partial pressure of oxygen; HCO$_3$ = bicarbonate.

Patient Outcomes

Patient will

- demonstrate normal or baseline gas exchange at rest and with exercise (see Table 5.5).
- respond to appropriate therapy and demonstrate no complications from oxygen administration, morphine sulfate, diuretics, vasodilators, and rotating tourniquets.

Nursing Interventions	Rationales
Assess for ongoing signs/symptoms of pulmonary congestion, including breathlessness, orthopnea, DOE, PND, nocturia, diaphoresis, cough, tachypnea, tachycardia, apprehension, decreased UO, weight gain, imbalanced I&O, elevated PCWP, hypoxemia, and hypercapnea.	Pulmonary congestion occurs when the left ventricle is no longer able to maintain forward blood flow, resulting in a backup of fluid in the pulmonary vasculature.
Assess for signs/symptoms of impaired gas exchange, including respiratory rate/rhythm, breath sounds, skin color/temperature, cyanosis, capillary refill time, ABGs, and cardiac rhythm.	Impaired gas exchange occurs as the fluid backs up first into the pulmonary vasculature, then into the alveoli, and finally into the larger airways, such as the bronchi.
Institute appropriate therapies for pulmonary vascular congestion/impaired, gas exchange, including	

Nursing Interventions	Rationales
1. oxygen	Supplemental oxygen is used when there is hypoxemia without severe hypercapnea. If arterial oxygen tension cannot be maintained at or near 60 mmHg with 100% oxygen or if progressive hypercapnia ensues, intubation and mechanical ventilation may be required.
2. high-Fowler's position, with legs dependent, if possible.	This position helps lower the diaphragm, increasing lung expansion and helps dilate peripheral arteries and veins, resulting in venous pooling of the blood. Dilating the peripheral arteries also reduces impedance to LV ejection, thus decreasing LVEDP.
3. morphine sulfate	Morphine sulfate reduces anxiety, decreases tachypnea, and causes peripheral pooling of the blood, thereby decreasing preload and afterload.
4. diuretics	Diuretics reduce total blood volume and prevent the recurrence of pulmonary congestion.
5. vasodilators	Vasodilators reduce SVR/PVR and thus enhance CO.
6. rotating tourniquets	Rotating tourniquets are only used if the above interventions have not worked to redistribute blood volume and decrease preload

NURSING DIAGNOSIS: FATIGUE

Related To limited cardiac reserve.

Defining Characteristics
Decreased mental and physical performance, speed, and capability
Impatience
Inaccuracy and increase in errors
Irritability
Listlessness

Loss of libido
Nervousness
Passivity
Tearfulness
Yawning

Patient Outcomes
Patient will
- learn to adjust activities to minimize fatigue.
- demonstrate an increased energy level.

Nursing Interventions	Rationales
Provide private room, when possible.	This reduces environmental stimuli contributing to fatigue.
Teach patient to count pulse before and after activities and record.	Pulse counting identifies activities which place high demands on the heart.
Space activities known to increase fatigue and schedule earlier in the day.	New activity should not be initiated until heart rate returns to preactivity level. Patients usually feel more rested earlier in the day.
Identify specific activities with which staff or family can assist.	

NURSING DIAGNOSIS: IMPAIRED PHYSICAL MOBILITY

Related To diminished cardiac output

Defining Characteristics
Decreased muscle strength, control, mass, or endurance
Impaired coordination
Impaired memory or intellectual capacity
Imposed restriction of movement due to a mechanical device or medical order
Inability to move purposefully within the physical environment
Limited range of motion
Reluctance to attempt movement

Patient Outcomes

Patient will
- not experience complications related to decreased mobility: skin breakdown, pulmonary problems, constipation, thromboembolism or phlebitis, depression, or confusion.
- participate in a supervised cardiac rehabilitation program.

Nursing Interventions	Rationales
Perform range-of-motion exercises and reposition patient every 2 hr.	Exercise improves muscular tone, aids venous return to the heart, and prevents skin breakdown and phlebitis.
Assist patient in coughing and deep-breathing exercises.	This prevents secondary pulmonary complications.
Apply antiembolic stockings and administer anticoagulant medications, if ordered.	Phlebitis and pulmonary emboli are common complictions of CHF.
Administer stool softeners and laxatives, as necessary. Use bedside commode.	Straining with bowel movements increases cardiac workload.
Provide emotional support, focusing on improvements in condition, assist with relaxation techniques, and encourage diversional activities.	Emotional upset can result in increased heart rate, SV, CO, blood pressure, and dysrhythmias at rest.
Explain need for bedrest and activity limitations.	Understanding need to minimize cardiac workload may decrease anxiety.
Explain cardiac rehabilitation and monitor response to progressive activity.	This provides direction and encouragement. Activity can be gradually increased based on hemodynamic tolerance.

NURSING DIAGNOSIS: ALTERED NUTRITION—LESS THAN BODY REQUIREMENTS

Related To anorexia, dyspnea, fatigue, and impaired absorption

Defining Characteristics

Body weight 20% or more under ideal for height and frame
Caloric intake (observed or reported) less than minimum daily requirement for current metabolic need

Decreased serum albumin
Decreased serum transferrin or iron-binding capacity
Decreased total protein
Electrolyte imbalance
Lack of interest in food
Poor skin turgor
Recent, unintentional weight loss of 20% or more of usual adult weight
Satiety immediately after ingesting small amounts of food
Weakness with loss of mobility

Patient Outcomes

Patient will maintain a positive nitrogen balance and stable weight within optimal range.

Nursing Interventions	Rationales
Assess nutritional status, including weight, appetite, and usual eating patterns.	Developing a plan that meets the nutritional needs and is acceptable to the patient, is based on an accurate collection of information.
Assess for factors that may alter gastrointestinal (GI) function.	Decreased activity and certain medications may slow GI motility. Constipation may cause feeling of abdominal fullness, thus decreasing appetite.
Conduct calorie count for 2–3 days.	A caloric intake summary provides objective data regarding the types and amounts of foods consumed.
Enlist patient assistance through discussion of food preferences and meal patterns.	Providing preferred foods and smaller, more frequent meals may aid in maintaining adequate nutritional intake.
Organize care to allow for 1-hr periods of rest before and after meals and maintain a quiet, relaxed environment.	Energy is conserved to minimize fatigue at mealtime.
Offer high-calorie, low-volume supplements between meals	Supplements allow ingestion of foods in small volumes with high nutrient density.
Encourage periods of exercise, as tolerated.	Exercise acts as an appetite stimulant and aids in digestion.

Nursing Interventions	Rationales
Instruct patient and family in specific nutritional needs, including restrictions.	Education is essential for understanding of individual needs and for follow-through with the nutritional program.

NURSING DIAGNOSIS: FEAR

Related To acute/chronic illness.

Defining Characteristics
Anger
Attends only to specific detail
Change in appetite
Change in sleep pattern
Chest tightness
Clinging
Crying
Difficulty in expressing self
Distractable
Dry mouth
Facial/muscle tension
Fatigue
Hyperventilation
Indecisive
Irritable
Palpitations
Selective inattention
Tachycardia
Trembling
Verbalizes/demonstrates inability to concentrate
Withdrawal

Patient Outcomes
Patient will
- verbalize feelings of anxiety/fear.
- use effective coping strategies throughout the course of the illness.
- demonstrate beneficial use of relaxation techniques.

Nursing Interventions	Rationales
Assess anxiety/fear, ask open-ended questions, and engage in active listening. Validate with patient.	These activities guide the patient in verbalizing stressors.

Nursing Interventions	Rationales
Sit with patient.	Focused attention conveys sincerity and interest, thus increasing the patient's comfort.
Use a therapeutic touch.	A therapeutic touch also enhances the patient's trust in the care provider.
Determine successful strategies used for coping with stress in the past and encourage use of these strategies.	Discussing past successes helps to focus patient on his or her strengths.
Encourage patient to interact and take an active role in daily care.	Including the patient in decision making increases his or her sense of purpose and reestablishes confidence.
Teach relaxation techniques, guided imagery, and music therapy.	Mastery of these techniques also helps to increase the patient's sense of control.
Give antianxiety medications, as needed.	Medication may be necessary in high-anxiety states.

NURSING DIAGNOSIS: KNOWLEDGE DEFICIT

Related To complex pathophysiological illness

Defining Characteristics
Inaccurate follow-through of instruction
Inadequate performance of demonstration of a skill
Inappropriate or exaggerated behaviors, for example, agitated, apathetic, hostile, hysterical
Lack of recall
Verbalizations indicating inadequate understanding, misinterpretation, or misconception of desired health behaviors

Patient Outcomes
Patient will verbalize knowledge of signs/symptoms of heart failure, risk factors/modification, medication regimen, activity level, diet, pulse counting, when to call physician for advice, and when to return for follow-up.

Nursing Interventions	Rationales
Assess needs and teach appropriate content regarding 1. signs/symptoms of heart failure 2. risk factor modification 3. medications 4. activity 5. diet 6. pulse counting 7. when to call for advice 8. when to return for follow-up	Effective teaching takes into account patient/family's readiness to learn, preexisting knowledge, phase of illness, and major concerns.

DISCHARGE PLANNING/CONTINUITY OF CARE

- Assist patient and family in coping with the immediate crisis of hospitalization.
- Provide support during the transition from intensive care to intermediate care.
- Assess home care environment and determine availability of needed social supports.
- Facilitate coordination of home care services, if required.
- Provide educational sessions for patient/family prior to discharge to facilitate compliance with home care treatment plan.

REFERENCES

Bousquet, G. L. (1990). Congestive heart failure: A review of nonpharmacological therapies. *Journal of Cardiovascular Nursing, 4*(3), 35–46.

Doyle, B. (1988). Nursing challenge: The patient with end-stage heart failure. In L. S. Kern (Ed.), *Cardiac critical care nursing* (pp. 311–356). Rockville, MD: Aspen.

Gettrust, K. V., & Brabec, P. D. (eds). (1992). *Nursing diagnosis in clinical practice*. Albany, NY: Delmar.

Moorhouse, M. S., Geissler, A. C., & Doenges, M. E. (1987). *Critical care plans*. Philadelphia: Davis.

Quaal, S. J. (1992). The person with heart failure and cardiogenic shock. In C. E. Guzzetta, & B. M. Dossey (Eds.), *Cardiovascular nursing—Holistic practice* (pp. 302–354). St. Louis, MO: Mosby Year Book.

Stanley, R. (1990). Drug therapy of heart failure. *Journal of Cardiovascular Nursing, 4*(3), 17–34.

Wright, S. M. (1990). Pathophysiology of congestive heart failure. *Journal of Cardiovascular Nursing: 4*(3), 1–16.

CARDIOGENIC SHOCK

Mary G. Schigoda, RN, MSN, CCRN

Cardiogenic shock is a complex clinical syndrome caused by inadequate delivery of blood to the major organs, particularly the heart, brain, and kidneys. It usually presents as a catastrophic complications of acute myocardial infarction (AMI) but can result from end-stage cardiac disease of any kind. Cardiogenic shock also may occur transiently after cardiac surgery. Despite technological and pharmacological advances in recent years, mortality still remains high due to a self-perpetuating cycle of progressive ischemic damage resulting in extensive, irreversible myocardial dysfunction.

ETIOLOGIES

- Myopathic factors (impaired myocardial contractility)
  - AMI, cardiomyopathy, cardiac amyloidosis, postoperative stunned myocardium
- Mechanical factors
  - Regurgitant lesions, that is, acute mitral or aortic insufficiency, ruptured intraventricular septum, or massive left ventricular (LV) aneurysm
  - Obstructive lesions of the LV outflow tract, that is, congenital/ acquired aortic stenosis or idiopathic hypertrophic subaortic stenosis (IHSS)
- Dysrhythmias
  - Brady/tachydysrhythmias and conduction disturbances

CLINICAL MANIFESTATIONS (see Table 6.1)

- Hypotension
- Tachycardia
- Impaired mentation/level of consciousness (LOC)
- Urine output (UO) < 30 mL/hr
- Peripheral vascular collapse

90

Table 6.1 • Clinical Manifestations Characterizing the Four Stages of Cardiogenic Shock

Stages of Shock	Clinical Manifestations
I: Initial stage	No signs or symptoms
II: Compensatory stage	Increased heart rate Cool, moist, pale skin Decreased urinary output Decreased peristalsis Increased rate/depth of respirations Pupillary dilation Altered level of consciousness
III: Progressive stage	Metabolic acidosis Edema (peripheral/pulmonary) Oliguria/anuria Decreased level of consciousness Hypotension Other organ failure
IV: Refractory stage	Worsening acidosis Further impaired respiratory and cerebral function and tissue perfusion Disseminated intravascular coagulation (DIC) Respiratory arrest Cardiac arrest Death

CLINICAL/DIAGNOSTIC FINDINGS

Noninvasive tests
- Electrocardiogram (ECG)
  - bradycardia/tachycardia
  - conduction defects
  - atrial/ventricular enlargement
  - LV aneurysm formation
  - ischemia/infarction
- Echocardiogram (ECHO)
  - atrial, ventricular, septal hypertrophy
  - valvular insufficiency/stenosis
  - septal and LV free wall motion abnormalities (akinesis, hypokinesis, paradoxical motion)
  - decreased LV ejection fraction (LVEF) <40%
- Chest x-ray (CXR)
  - cardiomegaly
  - pulmonary vascular congestion

- alveolar or interstitial edema
- pleural effusions
- Multigated blood pool imaging (MUGA) scan
  - wall motion abnormalities
  - decreased RVEF and/or LVEF
- Electrolytes
  - sodium (Na) low or high (due to renal dysfunction, fluid imbalance, and/or drug therapies
  - potassium (K) low or high (due to renal dysfunction, fluid imbalance, and/or drug therapies)
  - chloride (Cl) low or high (due to renal dysfunction, fluid imbalance, and/or drug therapies)
  - CO_2/HCO_3 low (metabolic acidosis due to decreased tissue perfusion)
- Renal function tests (RFTs)
  - blood urea nitrogen elevated
  - serum creatinine elevated
  - creatinine clearance low
- Liver function tests (LFTs)
  - lactate dehydrogenase (LDH) elevated
  - serum glutamic oxaloacetic transaminase/pyruvic transaminase (SGOT/SGPT) elevated
  - total bilirubin elevated
  - prothrombin time (PT) prolonged
- Complete blood count (CBC)
  - WBC (leukocytosis)
  - RBC (polycythemia)
  - Hgb/Hct (anemia)
- Clotting profile significantly altered (due to cellular damage)
- Arterial blood gases (ABGs) acid-base balance:
  - pH low (due to metabolic acidosis)
  - HCO_3 low (due to metabolic acidosis)
  - PaO_2 low (due to impaired oxygen transport)
  - $PaCO_2$ high (due to respiratory acidosis)
- Serum lactate levels elevated (due to poor perfusion and anaerobic metabolism)
- Cardiac enzymes elevated (with acute or recent MI)

Invasive tests
- Right-sided heart catheterization: demonstrates hemodynamic dysfunction, that is, high pulmonary artery pressure (PAP)/pulmonary capillary wedge pressure (PCWP)
- Left-sided heart catheterization: demonstrates hemodynamic dysfunction, that is, low LVEF, low cardiac output (CO)/cardiac index (CI)
- Coronary angiography: identifies coronary artery disease (CAD) induced ischemia/infarction as cause of shock

NURSING DIAGNOSIS: SEVERELY DECREASED CARDIAC OUTPUT

Related To compromised ventricular performance

Defining Characteristics
Abdominal distention
Abnormal heart sounds (S_3, S_4)
Angina
Crackles
Cyanosis; pallor of skin and mucous membranes
Decreased level of consciousness
Decreased peripheral pulses
Diaphoresis
Dyspnea
Dysrhythmias; other electrocardiographic changes
Edema (peripheral/pulmonary)
Ejection fraction < 40%
Elevated cardiac enzymes
Fatigue
Hypotension
Hypoxia
Jugular vein distension
Oliguria; anuria
Orthopnea
Shortness of breath
Weight gain

Patient Outcomes
Patient will
- demonstrate hemodynamic stability and increased ventricular performance, as evidenced by
  - hemodynamic parameters within normal limits (WNL) (see Table 5.1)
  - palpable pulses
  - respiratory rate 10–20 breaths per minute
  - warm, dry skin
  - urine output (UO) > 30 mL/hr
  - normal mentation and LOC; absence of restlessness, confusion, or psychosis
- demonstrate an increase in circulating blood volume following intravenous (IV) fluid challenge, as evidenced by
  - increased PAP and PCWP
- be free of pulmonary edema, as evidenced by
  - PCWP 15–20 mmHg
  - absence of dyspnea and orthopnea

- maintain satisfactory respiratory status and oxygenation.
- maintain a balanced intake & output (I&O).
- demonstrate increased CO and improved peripheral perfusion in response to sympathomimetic drugs.
- be free of dysrhythmias.
- demonstrate no complications from invasive hemodynamic monitoring, including
  - infection
  - dysrhythmias
  - pulmonary infarct
  - intact pulses distal to insertion site
  - normal sensation in extremity with monitoring line
- demonstrate no complications from the use of a ventricular assist device (VAD). (Refer to VADs.)

Nursing Interventions	Rationales
Evaluate hemodynamic stability and ventricular performance by assessing	Cardiogenic shock may progress through 4 stages as the condition deteriorates. (See Table 6.1.)
1. mean arterial pressure (MAP)	Circulating volume must be sufficient to maintain systolic blood pressure at 80–90 mmHg. Decreased pressure results in hypoperfusion of the myocardium exacerbating ischemia and further decreasing contractility.
2. CO/CI	Cardiac output measures cardiac function and is the product of heart rate and stroke volume (which is influenced by preload, afterload, and contractility). Cardiac index is a more specific determinant of CO, as it considers body size.
3. right atrial (RA) or central venous pressure (CVP)	Elevation suggests volume overload and/or heart failure (in the absence of volume overload).
4. PAP	Elevation reflects pulmonary congestion, indicative of heart failure.
5. PCWP	Elevation exceeding 16–18 mmHg reflects pulmonary congestion and left-sided heart failure.

Nursing Interventions	**Rationales**
6. heart rate and rhythm	Significant dysrhythmias may occur as the result of electrolyte/acid-base imbalances, catecholamines, drug toxicities, and hypoxemia, further decreasing coronary artery perfusion and increasing myocardial ischemia.
7. respiratory rate and effort (note use of accessory muscles)	Tachypnea or dyspnea may be the result of hypoxemia, acidosis, pulmonary edema, atelectasis, or pain.
8. skin color and temperature (note presence and quality of peripheral pulses)	Inadequate tissue perfusion is reflected by pallor, cyanosis, mottling, and cool, moist skin.
9. UO and specific gravity	Inadequate renal perfusion can result in acute tubular necrosis (ATN), with UO < 30 mL/hr and loss of ability to concentrate urine.
10. mentation/LOC	Inadequate cerebral perfusion may result in restlessness, confusion, lethargy, stupor, and coma.
11. bowel sounds (measure abdominal girth; note nausea, vomiting, pain; observe and guaiac nasogastric contents)	Inadequate mesenteric perfusion and/or inotropic drug therapy may alter gastrointestinal function, producing irritation, ischemia, pain, decrease/loss of peristalsis, and onset of ileus.
Monitor PAP/PCWP before, during, and after IV fluid challenges.	Intravenous fluids enhance circulating blood volume and increase left ventricular end-diastolic volume (LVEDV), which may increase contractility via Starling's law. Pulmonary capillary wedge pressure or pulmonary artery end-diastolic pressure determines whether the circulating volume needs to be expanded.

Nursing Interventions	Rationales
Monitor for signs of pulmonary edema: dyspnea, orthopnea, rales, and elevated PCWP.	Fluid in the pulmonary vasculature is indicated by a PCWP > 18 mmHg. The decreased distensibility of the lung increases the work of breathing, leading to dyspnea and orthopnea.
Evaluate respiratory status and oxygenation:	
1. Auscultate breath sounds.	The presence of rales, rhonchi, and wheezing may be indicative of fluid in the pulmonary vasculature.
2. Note peripheral or circumoral cyanosis.	Peripheral cyanosis reflects vasoconstriction and, to a lesser degree, hypoxemia. Central cyanosis is a more sensitive indicator of hypoxemia.
3. Maintain patent airway.	Suctioning may be needed to clear secretions and improve oxygen delivery.
4. Maintain bedrest, provide assistance with self-care needs, and schedule rest periods between activities/procedures.	This reduces oxygen needs/consumption.
5. Monitor ABGs.	Respiratory and metabolic acidosis may be present.
6. Provide supplemental oxygen.	Oxygen is needed to correct failing respiratory effort, hypoxemia, and acidosis.
Monitor hourly and 24-hr output and fluid volume.	Continuous IV fluid administration may potentiate volume overload, while the use of diuretics and oral fluid restrictions may deplete circulating volume
Administer sympathomimetic amines (dopamine, epinephrine, norepinephrine, isoproterenol, and neosynephrine) as prescribed, monitoring response (see Table 6.2).	Sympathomimetic amines increase myocardial contractility and reduce peripheral vascular resistance.

Nursing Interventions	**Rationales**
Assist in providing mechanical support for the failing heart.	Pharmacological agents are limited in their capacity to reduce myocardial oxygen demands and increase CO. Intra-aortic balloon pumps (IABPs) and ventricular assist devices (VADs) may partially or totally relieve the workload of the ventricles and potentially increase coronary artery perfusion. (Refer to VADs.)
Observe for complications related to hemodynamic monitoring lines, IABPs, and VADs.	Infection, dysrhythmias, pulmonary infarct, and circulatory compromise, particularly in the affected extremity, are potential complications related to hemodynamic monitoring, IABPs, and VADs. The risk of infection, however, may be even greater in this population due to the greatly decreased tissue perfusion.

NURSING DIAGNOSIS: FEAR

Related To severity of illness and threat of death

Defining Characteristics
Change in appetite
Change in sleep pattern
Chest tightness
Crying
Difficulty in expressing self
Facial/muscle tension
Fatigue
Hyperventilation
Indecisive
Irritable
Nausea/vomiting
Palpitations
Restlessness
Selective inattention
Tachycardia
Trembling
Verbalizes/demonstrates inability to concentrate
Withdrawal

Table 6.2 • Sympathomimetic Amines Commonly Used in the Treatment of Cardiogenic Shock

Drug	Usual IV Dosage	Dosage	Adrenergic Effects*		Comments
			Alpha	Beta	
Dopamine (intropin)	2–10 mcg/kg/min	Small Large	Minimal Marked	Minimal Moderate	Increased renal blood flow at <6 mcg/kg/min
Dobutamine (Dobutrex)	2.5–10.0 mcg/kg/min			Predominately stimulates myocardial β-receptors for inotropy.	Minimal chronotropic & peripheral vasoconstrictor effects.
Norepinephrine (Levophed)	2–8 mcg/min	Small Large	Moderate Marked	Minimal Moderate	May cause reflex slowing of HR due to increased BP.
Epinephrine (Adrenalin)	1–4 mcg/min	Small Large	Minimal Moderate	Moderate Marked	May cause tremors/anxiety.
Phenylephrine (Neo-Synephrine)	5–20 mcg/min		Predominantly stimulates alpha-receptors		
Isoproterenol (Isuprel)	2–20 mcg/min			Pure β-receptor stimulant.	May cause tremors/anxiety/dysrhythmias.

*alpha-adrenergic stimulation causes vasoconstriction, an increase in blood pressure, and further increase in afterload. beta-adrenergic stimulation causes a positive inotropic effect, reduces LVEDP, causes vasodilation, and reduces afterload.

Patient Outcomes

Patient will

- demonstrate an understanding of the need for continuous observation and anxiety management.
- verbalize (or otherwise communicate, if intubated) feelings of anxiety and fear of death.
- use effective coping strategies during course of illness.
- receive emotional/spiritual support from clergy and care providers.
- Family will communicate anxiety related to patient's illness to staff and verbalize fear of death.

Nursing Interventions	Rationales
Continue to reassess anxiety and provide ways to reduce fears.	Physiologically, the stress response results in high oxygen consumption, placing excessive demands on an already compromised heart.
Provide quiet environment.	A quiet environment minimizes external stimuli which may increase anxiety.
Explain all interventions.	Knowledge and understanding reduce anxiety/fear.
Use relaxation techniques.	These techniques are used to elicit the relaxation response which decreases sympathetic nervous system arousal, with resultant decrease in heart rate, respiratory rate, blood pressure, oxygen consumption, and anxiety. These techniques also promote feelings of peace and well-being.
Use guided imagery.	This promotes decreased stress and pain and helps redirect the patient toward healthy functioning as the desired effect.
Offer realistic reassurance.	Realistic reassurance promotes trust in care providers.

Nursing Interventions	Rationales
Provide for uninterrupted time for patient/family to communicate feelings.	Communication may be more laborious if patient is intubated. Focusing on the family unit conveys sincerity and builds trust.
Encourage use of previously successful coping strategies.	Encouraging the use of previously successful coping focuses on strengths.
Allow time for patient/family to express fear of death.	Allowing time for discussion of death conveys compassion. The venting of difficult emotions can be cathartic, which can promote healing in someone experiencing emotional/spiritual distress.
If death is eminent, stay with the patient and family to assist them.	Often the patient and/or family have not experienced death in such a personal manner. The uncertainty of what to expect may make them apprehensive of being alone. Being with them during this time conveys caring and may reduce unrealistic fears.
Provide emotional/spiritual support for patient/family by	
1. allowing family to be with patient for extended periods of time	The patient and family may derive great comfort and support from each other during this time of great need.
2. use of presence	Being present for the patient and family promotes mutual sharing and demonstrates the nurse's commitment.
3. encouraging reminiscence and life review	Through reminiscence and life review persons often can resolve or come to understand certain life situations from a new perspective. It provides an opportunity to "let go" of aspects of oneself and to grieve for losses.

Nursing Interventions	Rationales
4. use of prayer	Many patients and families have expressed the helpfulness of prayer, particularly in times of crisis. Nurses may be asked to pray with, pray for, or remain with the patient during a prayer.
5. calling clergy, if requested	Clergy can be helpful when the situation requires more in-depth or long-term follow-up than the nurse can provide.

DISCHARGE PLANNING/CONTINUITY OF CARE

- Wean inotropic and/or mechanical support as tolerated.
- Recognize and treat further complicating problems.
- Assist the patient in achieving a peaceful death.

REFERENCES

Bousquet, G. L. (1990). Congestive heart failure: A review of nonpharmacologic therapies. *Journal of Cardiovascular Nursing, 4*(3), 35–46.

Gettrust, K. V. & Brabec, P. D. (1992). *Nursing diagnosis in clinical practice*. Albany, NY: Delmar.

Quaal, S. J. (1992). The person with heart failure and cardiogenic shock. In C. E. Guzzetta & B. M. Dossey (Eds.), *Cardiovascular nursing— Holistic practice* (pp. 302–354). St. Louis, MO: Mosby Year Book.

Stanley, R. (1990). Drug therapy of heart failure. *Journal of Cardiovascular Nursing, 4*(3), 17–34.

Wright, S. M. (1990). Pathophysiology of congestive heart failure. *Journal of Cardiovascular Nursing, 4*(3), 1–16.

CARDIOMYOPATHY AND MYOCARDITIS

Maurice H. Espinoza RN, MSN

Cardiomyopathy is a debilitating form of heart disease which results from deterioration of the heart muscle. A number of forms of cardiomyopathy are seen, including structural, hypertrophic, and dilated cardiomyopathy. In the critical care unit the dilated form of cardiomyopathy is seen most commonly. This form of cardiomyopathy strikes young and old alike and both sexes. Dilated cardiomyopathy can develop after a viral disease, develop from end-stage coronary artery disease (ischemic cardiomyopathy), or be idiopathic. The cardiac muscle fibers contract poorly, causing progressive global left ventricular dysfunction manifested by dysrhythmias, low cardiac output, and eventually refractory congestive heart failure.

ETIOLOGIES

- Viral infections
- End-stage coronary artery disease
- Valvular heart disease
- Congenital heart disease
- Alcoholism
- Pregnancy (peripartum cardiomyopathy)
- Cancer chemotherapy
- Immunological disorders
- Idiopathic
- Familial

CLINICAL MANIFESTATIONS

There is often a long latency period during which the myocardial function deteriorates. Symptoms usually go undetected until the symptoms of congestive heart failure are seen. Many of the diagnostic findings will be the same as those seen in congestive heart failure:

- fatigue
- dyspnea
- increased heart rate
- weight gain
- dysrhythmias
- jugular venous distention
- ascites
- dry cough
- palpitations
- anorexia
- edema
- S_3 gallop
- hepatomegaly
- diaphoresis

CLINICAL/DIAGNOSTIC FINDINGS

Electrocardiogram (ECG)
- Ventricular ectopy associated with ventricular enlargement.
- Atrial fibrillation associated with atrial enlargement

Chest x-ray
- Cardiomegaly
- Increased interstitial markings consistent with congestive heart failure.

Endomyocardial biopsy
- Confirms suspected cellular abnormalities
- Diagnoses systemic conditions such as amyloidosis, sarcoidosis

Echocardiogram
- Dilated atrial and ventricular chambers
- Global hypokinesis to akinesis of ventricles
- Decreased ejection fraction due to decrease in wall motion
- Valvular insufficiency due to dilated heart
- Mural thrombi

MUGA scan (multigated blood pool imaging scan)
- Dilation of both atria
- Dilation of both ventricles
- Global hypokinesis to akinesis of ventricles
- Decreased ejection fraction of both ventricles

Cardiac catheterization
- Pulmonary hypertension
- Documents coronary anatomy: normal coronary arteries or narrowing of coronary arteries in ischemic cardiomyopathy
- Low left ventricular ejection fraction

Electrolytes
- Na—hyponatremia, dilutional or due to diuretics
- K— hyperkalemia, due to renal insufficiency; hypokalemia, due to diuretics
- Cl— hypochloremia, dilutional or due to diuretics

Renal function tests
Decreased perfusion of the kidneys causes renal insufficiency:
- BUN—elevated, due to poor renal perfusion
- creatinine—elevated, due to poor renal perfusion
- urinalysis—elevated specific gravity

Liver function tests
As with CHF, levels will be elevated due to passive liver congestion:
- Lactate dehydrogenase (LDH) elevated
- Serum glutamic oxaloacetic/pyruvic transaminase (SGOT/SGPT) elevated
- total bilirubin elevated

MYOCARDITIS

Myocarditis can be described as an inflammation of the cardiac muscle. The disease can affect the pericardium and the ventricles. Myocardial involvement may be focal or diffuse. Myocarditis has two stages, an acute stage where necrosis occurs from virus-induced myocyte destruction and a chronic stage where autoimmune mediated myocyte destruction occurs. The acute stage occurs at 5–7 days, with the chronic stage occurring 9–45 days later. Patients may recover from myocarditis or go on to develop dilated cardiomyopathy.

ETIOLOGIES

- Viral infections—coxsackievirus A and B strains, echovirus, poliovirus, influenza, rubeola, rubella
- Bacterial infections—tuberculosis, tetanus, diphtheria, staphylococcal, pneumococcal and gonococcal infections
- Parasitic infections—trypanosomiasis, toxoplasmosis
- Helminthic infections—trichinosis
- Hypersensitive immune response—acute rheumatic fever
- Radiation therapy—large doses of radiation to chest in treating lung or other cancers
- Chemical poisons—alcohol

CLINICAL MANIFESTATIONS

Clinical manifestations of myocarditis may be nonspecific, and the diagnosis of myocarditis may be difficult to document. Patients present with a wide variety of symptoms:
- easy fatigability
- pericardial pain
- pericardial rub
- fever
- exertional dyspnea
- syncope
- heart failure

CLINICAL/DIAGNOSTIC FINDINGS

The diagnostic testing related to myocarditis has little specificity pertaining to myocarditis and is done to rule out other causes associated with the clinical manifestations.

Laboratory values
- Elevated white blood cell count
- Elevated erythrocyte sedimentation rate
- Cardiac enzymes elevated: [creatine phosophokinase (CPK), CPK isoenzymes, serum glutamic pyruvic transaminase (SGOT), lactic dehydrogenase]
- Elevated antibody titers

Electrocardiogram
- Typically shows diffuse ST-segment and T-wave abnormalities
- Conduction changes—prolonged PR interval
  - atrial or ventricular dysrhythmias
  - atrioventricular conduction changes
  - bundle branch block
  - complete heart block

Gallium scan
The radioisotope is taken up in the inflamed myocardium. A positive scan is tentative support that myocarditis is present.

Chest x-ray
- Pleural effusion
- Cardiomegaly
- Increased interstitial markings

Culture of body fluids
Demonstration of the presence of a virus is supportive but not conclusive for myocarditis.

Endomyocardial biopsy
This may be the only definitive clinical method of diagnosing myocarditis. When the usual five samples of tissue are taken via right-sided heart catheterization, the sensitivity for myocarditis may be as low as 50%.

NURSING DIAGNOSIS: DECREASED CARDIAC OUTPUT

Related To decreased myocardial contractility

Defining Characteristics

Hypotension
Fatigue
Oliguria
Rales
Restlessness
Syncope
Cough
Gallop rhythm

Dysrhythmias
Jugular venous distention
Cold clammy skin
Orthopnea
Shortness of breath (SOB)
Vertigo
Weakness

Patient Outcomes

- Adequate cardiac output will be maintained as evidenced by stable blood pressure (mean arterial blood pressure > 90) and acceptable hemodynamics (cardiac index > 2.0)

- The number of life-threatening dysrythmias will decrease as evidenced by stable electrocardiogram (ECG).
- The skin will be warm and dry.
- Urine output will be at least 30 mL/hr.
- The sensorium will be clear.

Nursing Interventions	Rationales
Assess level of consciousness.	Changes in cardiac output may be first seen as changes in sensorium, such as confusion or restlessness.
Monitor complete hemodynamics (see Table 7.1): central venous pressure (CVP), pulmonary artery pressure (PAP), pulmonary capillary wedge pressure (PCWP), cardiac output (CO) and cardiac index (CI), systemic vascular resistance (SVR), and pulmonary vascular resistance (PVR).	Hemodynamic parameters must be monitored when titrating inotropic and vasodilating medications. These agents enhance cardiac contractility and decrease vascular resistance, facilitating left ventricular emptying and making it easier for the heart to pump effectively. Optimal manipulation of hemodynamics will improve perfusion of vital organs.
Administer inotropic medications that will help improve cardiac output: 1. dobutamine 2. norepinephrine 3. dopamine 4. amrinone 5. digoxin	These pharmacological agents improve cardiac output and improve perfusion to vital organs. All medications which improve cardiac function will increase the workload of the myocardium, and possible adverse effects of these medications must be monitored closely.
Administer pharmacological agents that will reduce systemic and pulmonary vascular resistance, thereby decreasing the workload of the heart: 1. nitroprusside 2. angiotensin converting enzyme (ACE) inhibitors—enalapril, captopril 3. beta blockers 4. hydralazine 5. prostaglandin E_1 6. nitroglycerin	Vasodilating agents open the vessels wider, allowing the heart to pump against a lower resistance. Again, side effects of pharmacological agents must be considered when choosing an afterload reducing agent. All may cause hypotension. In addition, nitroprusside may cause thyocynate toxicity. The ACE inhibitors are used cautiously in renal insufficiency.

Nursing Interventions	Rationales
Monitor oxygenation via pulse oximetry or arterial blood gases.	An adequate supply of oxygen will improve cardiac function and will help decrease lactic acidosis resulting from anaerobic metabolism.
Monitor respiratory pattern.	Changes in depth or rate may signify pulmonary congestion.
Assess complaint of shortness of breath quickly.	This is often the first sign of impending congestive heart failure.
Monitor urine output.	Urine output is a reflection of cardiac output, as it is related to perfusion of the kidneys.
Control dysrhythmias promptly by administering antidysrhythmic agents as prescribed.	With cardiomyopathy and myocarditis, conduction changes in the diseased myocardium may lead to lethal dysrhythmias.
Monitor drug levels of antidysrhythmic agents: lidocaine, procainamide, bretylium, amiodarone, and mexilitene.	Levels of these medications should be monitored to ensure therapeutic levels and avoid toxic effects.
Administer anticoagulants as prescribed.	Mural thrombi may form in the hypocontractile heart, predisposing to thromboembolism.
Limit activity during periods of low cardiac output.	Activity increases oxygen demand, which must be met by increased uptake in the tissues and increased oxygen delivery by the heart. This increased demand places a greater workload on the heart and may cause a greater oxygen need than can be provided. This oxygen mismatch may lead to dysrhythmias and other adverse side effects such as hypotension and shortness of breath.

Table 7.1 • Hemodynamic Parameters

Parameter	Normal Measurement	Hemodynamic Significance
CVP: pressure in right atrium	0–5 mmHg	Elevated CVP indicates volume overload. Increased venous return and elevated CVP may lead to right ventricular failure
PAP: pressure in pulmonary artery	15–25/8–15 mmHg	Increased PAP pressures reflect overall fluid accumulation. Increased PAD reflects PCWP.
PCWP: pressure in left atrium	6–12 mmHg	Elevated PCWP indicates decreased left ventricular function and increased pooling of blood in lungs.
CO: heart rate × stroke volume	4–8 L/min	Decreased CO indicates decreased myocardial contractility and perfusion
CI: CO/body surface area	2.5–3.5 L/min/m²	<2.0 cell damage begins to occur from decreased perfusion
SVR: [(MAP − CVP)/CO] × 80	800–1200 dyn/s/cm^{-5}	Increased SVR causes increased myocardial workload on left side of heart and decreased perfusion to body.
PVR: [(Mean PAP − PCWP)/CO] × 80	150–250 dyn/s/cm^{-5}	Elevated PVR causes increased myocardial workload on right side of heart and decreased perfusion to lungs.

Note: CVP = central venous pressure, PAP = pulmonary artery pressure, PCWP = pulmonary capillary wedge pressure, CO = cardiac output, CI = cardiac index, SVR = systemic vascular resistance, MAP = mean arterial pressure, PAP = pulmonary artery pressure

▼

NURSING DIAGNOSIS: ALTERED TISSUE PERFUSION—PERIPHERAL AND RENAL

Related To decreased arterial blood flow

Defining Characteristics

Capillary refill time > 3 s
Edema
Mottling
Decreased urine output

Cyanosis
Increased tissue turgor
Cold clammy skin

Patient Outcomes

The patient will demonstrate adequate peripheral and renal tissue perfusion, as evidenced by

- a balanced intake and output
- absence of peripheral edema
- presence of palpable peripheral pulses
- warm, dry extremities
- vital signs within the patient's normal range
- urine output ≥30 mL/hr

Nursing Interventions	Rationales
Asses capillary refill, skin color, temperature, and strength of peripheral pulses.	Peripheral vasoconstriction will decrease the amount of blood flow to the extremities in exchange for increased blood flow to core of the body.
Assess blood pressure frequently.	A mean arterial blood pressure greater than 90 mmHg is necessary to supply basic perfusion to the kidneys.
Assess urine output for amount, color, concentration.	Changes in the amount of urine may signify a drop in perfusion to the kidneys. Changes in appearance and color may indicate changes in renal perfusion pressure and decrease in the glomerular filtration rate.

Nursing Interventions	Rationales
Monitor laboratory values indicative of renal function closely: potassium, sodium, creatinine, and blood urea nitrogen (BUN).	Rising creatinine and BUN demonstrate renal insufficiency. A rising serum potassium may also occur. Electrolyte depletion is common when loop diuretics are used; replacement therapy may be indicated.
Administer renal dose dopamine as ordered.	Renal dose dopamine (2–5 μg/kg/min) dilates the mesenteric arteries, increasing blood flow to the renal arteries and providing better perfusion to the kidneys. High-dose dopamine decreases blood flow to the kidneys.
Administer dobutamine to maintain adequate cardiac output.	In cardiomyopathy and myocarditis, the cardiac output diminishes and may not supply adequate perfusion to the vital organs. Dobutamine is a selective agent which stimulates the heart to pump more effectively increasing flow to the kidneys.

NURSING DIAGNOSIS: FLUID VOLUME EXCESS

Related To decreased glomular filtration

Defining Characteristics

Peripheral edema
Weight gain
Orthopnea
Pulmonary congestion
Decrease in blood pressure
Increased pulmonary artery pressure
Oliguria

Pleural and pericardial effusion
Shortness of breath
S_3 heart sound
Rales
Increased central venous pressure
Jugular venous distention

Patient Outcomes

- Fluid balance will be maintained, as evidenced by stable weight and balanced intake and output.
- Adequate oxygenation will be maintained, as evidenced by a normal acid/base balance and pulse oxymetry above 92%.
- Peripheral edema will decrease.

- Jugular venous distention will decrease, as evidenced by a lowered CVP (<10 mmHg).
- Adequate urine output above 30 mL/hr will be maintained.

Nursing Interventions	Rationales
Monitor intake/output and daily weight.	Adequacy of hydration and trends in fluid balance are assessed by these values.
Assess respiratory rate and character, pulse oximetry, and arterial blood gases.	As pulmonary congestion increases, respiratory distress may develop from pulmonary edema and may require intubation to provide adequate oxygenation.
Assess peripheral edema state.	As the urine output decreases, more fluid is retained in the body, leading to venous congestion and peripheral edema.
Administer diuretics as ordered.	Diuretics will decrease fluid retention and edema. Larger doses of diuretics may be required to reach the desired effect.
Administer electrolyte replacement as ordered.	Replacement of electrolytes will be needed when loop diuretics are used. However, replacement therapy should be initiated cautiously with decreased renal function.
Provide low-sodium diet.	A diet low in sodium will allow more free water to be excreted through the kidneys and will decrease the amount of peripheral edema.
Concentrate intravenous (IV) medications to minimize IV fluid intake.	Concentrating the solution will allow less free water to be administered when inotropes and antidysrhythmic drugs are administered. A less concentrated solution may be used when weaning the medications.

NURSING DIAGNOSIS: ALTERED NUTRITION—LESS THAN BODY REQUIREMENTS

Related To anorexia and fatigue

Defining Characteristics
Loss of weight
Aversion to eating
Perceived inability to ingest food
Poor muscle tone
Reported inadequate food intake
Lack of interest in food

Patient Outcomes
- Stable weight will be maintained.
- Adequate intake will be maintained, as evidenced by normal nutritional parameters.
- Nutritional intake will be appropriate to body energy requirements and expenditures.

Nursing Interventions	Rationales
Measure and document oral intake by conducting a calorie count.	Patients with symptoms of heart failure are often unable to maintain adequate nutritional intake.
Weigh daily at the same time in similar clothing.	A general trend in weight gain or loss can be documented.
Monitor laboratory values indicative of nutritional state: electrolytes, magnesium, phosphorus, calcium, albumin, total protein, and serum cholesterol.	Electrolyte abnormalities may occur with hypertonic enteral feedings displaying the need for hydration or electrolyte replacement. Other values may decrease if feedings are not being adequately absorbed.
Monitor for signs or symptoms of infection: inflammation at IV sites, temperature > 100 °F, shaking chills, and increased white blood cell (WBC) count.	Inadequate nutrition predisposes the patient to immunosuppresion, increasing the possibility of infection.
Initiate dietary consult and in collaboration with the clinical dietitian perform nitrogen balance studies.	Nitrogen excretion may be greater than intake, representing a negative nitrogen balance and breakdown of proteins for energy.

Nursing Interventions	**Rationales**
Offer diet high in protein and in small portions frequently.	This will ensure that the patient keep adequate blood protein levels and not break down muscle protein for energy.
Allow adequate rest periods between meals.	Allowing adequate rest will help the patient to have enough to eat, thereby increasing caloric intake.
Provide enteral nutrition early if patient is unable to eat orally.	Early treatment will decrease weight loss and protein breakdown.

NURSING DIAGNOSIS: ANXIETY

Related To life-threatening cardiac compromise

Defining Characteristics
Subjective
- Increased tension
- Uncertainty
- Fearfulness
- Changes in life events
- Anxiousness

Objective
- Cardiovascular excitation
- Superficial vasoconstriction
- Pupil dilation
- Restlessness
- Hand tremors
- Facial tension
- Increased perspiration

Patient Outcomes
- Feelings of anxiety will be verbalized.
- Sources of anxiety will be identified.
- Positive problem-solving skills will be demonstrated.
- Methods of social and professional support are identified and utilized.
- Decrease in anxiety will be demonstrated both verbally and behaviorally.

Nursing Interventions	Rationales
Assess the need for information and provide accurate information in a variety of ways in simple to understand language.	Assessment of knowledge and readiness to receive information is as important as the information given. The critically ill may not be ready for detailed information but appreciate simple explanations.
Inform patient of tests and procedures.	Information given prior to the procedure will allow for clarification of any misconceptions and an opportunity to answer any questions.
Identify feelings and encourage verbalization.	Verbalization of feelings will allow concerns to be recognized and lead to more effective problem solving.
Identify anxiety-producing situations.	Staff may then avoid unnecessary anxiety-producing situations. If unable to avoid them, a plan to help the patient and family deal with them can be arranged.
Keep family informed of patient's condition and allow for extended visiting.	Keeping the family informed will facilitate better understanding of problems and treatment and also enhance communication between staff and family members. This communication is the basis for the trust which must develop between staff and family. Extended visiting should be encouraged when the patient response to the visiting is positive. For the most part, family members are better able to help the patient deal with the cardiomyopathy.
Identify problem-solving skills and past methods of coping.	In identifying these skills the nurse will empower the patient to rely on existing strategies for dealing with stress.

▼

DISCHARGE PLANNING/CONTINUITY OF CARE

- Begin discharge planning near the end of the critical care stay when the patient is hemodynamically stable.
- Identify resources that will be needed at home, such as oxygen or complex medication administration, and briefly discuss with the family. Allow time for family preparedness and encourage family involvement.
- Document information already shared with the patient and family so teaching can be reinforced and continued after transfer from the critical care unit.

REFERENCES

Bohachick, P., & Anton, B. (1990). Psychosocial adjustment of patients and spouses to severe cardiomyopathy. *Research in Nursing and Allied Health, 13,* 385–392.

Grady, K. L., & Costanzo-Nordin, M. R. (1989). Myocarditis: A review of a clinical enigma. *Heart & Lung, 18*(4), 347–353.

McNulty, C. M. (1992). Active viral myocarditis: Application of current knowledge to clinical practice. *Heart Disease and Stroke, 1,* 135–140.

Owens-Jones, S., & Hopp, L. (1988). Viral myocarditis. *Focus on Critical Care, 15*(1), 25–37.

Purcell, J. A., Holder, K. (1989). Cardiomyopathy: Understanding the problem. *American Journal of Nursing, 89*(1), 57–74, 74b.

Vitello-Cicciu, J. (1987). Nursing grand rounds—the patient with viral cardiomyopathy. *Journal of Cardiovascular Nursing, 2*(1), 48–52.

▼

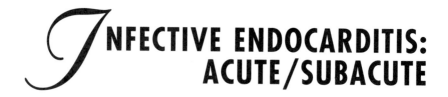

INFECTIVE ENDOCARDITIS: ACUTE/SUBACUTE

Julie A. Sommer, RN, MSN

Infective endocarditis is an infectious and inflammatory condition involving the heart valves and endothelial lining of the heart. It remains a serious illness associated with high mortality in spite of modern antimicrobial therapy. Infective endocarditis can lead to a variety of physiological problems. In addition to febrile illness and cardiac complications, cerebral infarction, renal failure, pulmonary emboli, and unilateral blindness may occur. With a variety of signs and symptoms, diagnosis can be difficult.

The most common feature of infective endocarditis is the appearance of vegetations on the cardiac valve leaflets. These vegetations develop through different mechanisms in the acute and subacute forms of the disease. Acute infective endocarditis results when normal heart valves become infected with a highly virulent organism. It has a rapid onset and left untreated results in extensive cardiac damage, morbidity, and mortality within days to weeks. Subacute infective endocarditis commonly occurs in persons with congenital or acquired valvular cardiac lesions following dental or medical procedures. Bacteria considered to be normal flora adhere to the abnormal perivalvular tissue and begin an insidious infection. It has a gradual onset and is more likely to be treated successfully than acute endocarditis.

ETIOLOGIES

- Systemic bacteremia
  - Acute endocarditis: group A nonhemolytic *Streptococcus*, *pneumococcus*, and *staphylococcus*
  - Subacute endocarditis: *Streptococcus viridans* and *S. faecalis*.
- Intravenous drug use
- Poor oral hygiene
- Trauma to skin integrity
- Dental procedures
- Invasive monitoring and procedures
  - cardiac catheterization
  - cardiac valve surgery

- transvenous pacing
- gastrointestinal (GI) and genitourinary (GU) procedures
- intravenous lines

CLINICAL MANIFESTATIONS

Infectious process
- Flulike symptoms
- Low-grade fever
- Anorexia
- Weight loss
- Weakness
- Chills
- Sweats
- Myalgias
- Arthralgias

Cardiac involvement
- Heart murmur
- Heart failure
- Conduction changes
- Pericarditis and myocarditis
- Embolization of vegetations can result in vascular occlusions and infarctions of
  - brain
  - kidney
  - spleen
  - heart
  - eye
  - gut
  - lungs
  - vertebral arteries
- Mycotic aneurysms: a localized abnormal expansion of a vessel due to destruction of part or all of its wall by microorganisms.

Immunological response
- Allergic vasculitis
  - petechiae
  - splinter hemorrhages
  - Janway lesions: flat, painless, erythematous lesions, 1–4 mm in diameter, on the palms, soles, and extremities
  - Roth's spots: lesions on the sclera and retina that are circular or flame shaped
  - Osler's nodes: small reddened, painful nodules with white centers, located on the terminal phalanges, palms, soles, and lower arms

CLINICAL/DIAGNOSTIC FINDINGS

Laboratory Tests
- Elevated white blood (WBC) count
- Positive blood cultures: three sets of aerobic and anaerobic blood cultures may be necessary to isolate the organism
- Elevated erythrocyte sedimentation rate
- Normochromic, normocytic anemia
- Elevated rheumatoid factor
- Presence of circulating immune complexes

Two-dimensional echocardiography
Identifies and evaluates the degree of valvular destruction and the presence, size, and mobility of vegetations.

NURSING DIAGNOSIS: INFECTIVE THERMOREGULATION

Related To infection

Defining Characteristics
Temperature > 101.5 °F
Shaking chills

Patient Outcomes
The patient will be free of infection, as evidenced by
- body temperature < 100 °F
- negative blood cultures

Nursing Interventions	Rationales
Record temperature hourly. If afebrile, increase interval to every 2–4 hr.	The most common feature of infective endocarditis is fever. This feature may be absent in the elderly because of an impaired immune response.
If fever is present, assess for signs and symptoms of dehydration: dry mucous membranes, poor skin turgor, and excessive thirst.	Fever increases water loss via the skin and lungs.
Record daily weight and intake and output.	Weight loss and negative fluid balance may indicate dehydration.

Nursing Interventions	Rationales
Obtain initial serial blood cultures prior to beginning antimicrobial therapy. Obtain subsequent cultures at intervals throughout the course of antimicrobial therapy.	Blood cultures are necessary to isolate the causative organism. Once antimicrobial therapy is started, blood cultures evaluate the effectiveness of microbial therapy.
Before initiating antimicrobial therapy, determine the patient's allergy history. During the course of therapy observe and document allergic reactions and any adverse effects of therapy: penicillin reactions (mild rashes, hives, urticaria, fever, diarrhea, anaphylactic shock); vancomycin and gentamycin (nephrotoxicity, ototoxicity, fever, and mild rashes).	Commonly used antibiotics can produce allergic and adverse reactions.
Administer broad-spectrum intravenous (IV) antibiotics as prescribed initially and adjust according to the organism identified via blood cultures.	Antibiotic therapy is usually prescribed for 6–8 weeks because of the adherence properties of the bacteria deep within the vegetations.
Obtain peak and trough levels after the third dose of antibiotics and periodically during antibiotic therapy.	The goal of antibiotic therapy is to provide therapeutic serum drug levels and minimize drug side effects. Additionally, the elderly and others may require lower drug dosages secondary to slower detoxification through the liver and kidneys.
Observe IV site for signs of warmth, redness, swelling, or drainage. Promptly discontinue the IV when infection or infiltration is suspected. Change IV site every 48–72 hr or according to the hospital policy for IV lines.	If infection is suspected, the IV catheter is changed to limit the chance of further sepsis.
Facilitate insertion of a long-term IV catheter.	Long-term catheters can easily provide dependable IV access in both inpatient and outpatient settings.

NURSING DIAGNOSIS: HIGH RISK FOR DECREASED CARDIAC OUTPUT

Risk Factors
- Valvular insufficiency
- Cardiac abscesses
- Congestive heart failure
- Myocardial infarction

Patient Outcomes
Stable cardiac output will be maintained, as evidenced by
- heart rate and rhythm within normal parameters
- systolic blood pressure > 90 mmHg
- clear lungs on auscultation
- normal arterial blood gases (ABGs) or pulse oximetry > 92%

Nursing Interventions	Rationales
Auscultate the heart and report any new murmurs and changes in the sound of old murmurs.	A common finding in infective endocarditis is a murmur, from valvular destruction.
Assess for signs and symptoms of left-sided heart failure: S_3 gallop, cough, sporadic dyspnea, hypotension, narrowed pulse pressure, cool clammy skin, pulmonary edema, and difficulty concentrating.	Vegetations most frequently destroy the mitral or aortic valves causing left-sided heart failure.
Monitor vital signs and hemodynamics: central venous pressure (CVP), pulmonary artery pressure (PAP), pulmonary capillary wedge pressure (PCWP), cardiac output (CO), and cardiac index (CI).	Valvular insufficiency creates a gradual decrease in the forward flow of blood through the heart, raising pulmonary vascular resistance and decreasing cardiac output. As the heart begins to decompensate, a cascade of events follow, resulting in decreased blood pressure and increased CVP, PAP, and PCWP, with further deterioration of CO.
Assess and report (electrocardiogram (ECG) conduction changes.	Septal abscesses or myocarditis may cause conduction abnormalities.

Nursing Interventions	**Rationales**
Monitor ECG and report abnormal Q-wave and ST-segment deviations	Myocardial infarction (MI) can occur if an embolic vegetation occludes a major coronary artery.
Monitor and report frequency, location, intensity, duration, and type of chest pain suggestive of MI: 1. continuous pain 2. radiation to neck, jaw, back, arms 3. nausea, vomiting, abdominal discomfort 4. diaphoresis	Early recognition of MI can lead to early treatment to prevent complications.
Obtain serial enzymes as ordered and monitor the results.	Intracellular enzymes, creatinine phosphokinase (CPK), cardiac isoenzymes, and lactate dehydrogenase (LDH) are released into the blood during MI.
Record intake and output and daily weight and report a 3-lb weight gain in 24 hr.	Abnormal increases in extracellular fluid retention occurs in congestive heart failure
Maintain prescribed fluid restriction.	Increased fluid puts increased work on the heart, causing congestive heart failure.
Administer oxygen and monitor ABGs and pulse oximetry to evaluate effective oxygenation.	Oxygenation is impaired by pulmonary vascular congestion secondary to left ventricular failure.
Elevate head of bed.	Elevating the head of bed decreases the work of breathing by allowing gravity to pull the diaphragm and abdominal contents downward, providing for greater thoracic expansion.

NURSING DIAGNOSIS: HIGH RISK FOR ALTERED TISSUE PERFUSION

Risk Factors
- Mycotic emboli
  - cerebral emboli
  - abdominal or thoracic emboli
  - pulmonary emboli
  - renal emboli

Patient Outcomes
The patient will be free of the symptoms of systemic embolizations, as evidenced by
- absence of neurological deficits
- absence of thoracic or abdominal pain
- absence of dyspnea

Nursing Interventions	Rationales
Assess for signs and symptoms of cerebral embolization: changes in level of consciousness, sudden localized headache, seizures, transient weakness, numbness or tingling on one side, hemiplegia, aphasia, and visual field defects.	The most common neurological complication of infective endocarditis is cerebral embolization. In addition, cerebral mycotic aneurysms are manifested by persistent localized headaches, central nervous system complaints, and visual field defects.
Assess and report complaints of thoracic, abdominal, and back pain.	Abdominal or thoracic mycotic aneurysms can develop as a complication. Symptoms may include backache from the occlusion of a vertebral vessel and left upper quadrant pain from infarction of the spleen.
Assess for signs and symptoms of pulmonary embolization: decreased PaO_2, dyspnea, sudden chest or shoulder pain, hemoptysis, nonproductive cough, anxiety, restlessness, hypotension, and tachycardia and pulmonary infiltrates on chest x-ray.	Endocarditis can lead to pulmonary emboli from vegetative embolization.

NURSING DIAGNOSIS: ACTIVITY INTOLERANCE

Related To infection, cardiac decompensation, and imposed bedrest

Defining Characteristics

Verbal report of fatigue or weakness during or following activity
Crackles auscultated in lung fields
Dyspnea on exertion
Postural hypotension
Tremors
Loss of muscle strength.

Patient Outcomes

- Activity level will increase
- The patient will be free of complications of prolonged bedrest, as evidenced by
  - clear breath sounds on auscultation
  - adequate muscle tone
  - intact skin over bony prominences

Nursing Interventions	Rationales
Perform respiratory assessment with each vital sign check. Note signs of atelectasis such as dyspnea and decreased breath sounds.	Atelectasis is a common complication of prolonged bedrest and contributes to the development of pneumonia.
Assist with coughing and deep breathing every 2 hr.	Coughing and deep breathing mobilize secretions and decrease atelectasis.
Perform passive range-of-motion exercises every 4 hr while awake. Progress to active range-of-motion exercises as tolerated.	Joint mobility and muscle tone is maintained through passive and active exercises. Pain from endocarditis complications may limit mobility.
Turn every 2 hours.	Frequent position changes provide comfort and prevent skin breakdown secondary to bedrest.
Massage skin to prominent areas or potential breakdown areas with each turn.	
Provide scheduled rest periods between activities.	Fatigue is common secondary to fever, altered cardiac output, and anemia.

Nursing Interventions	Rationales
Assist with eating, bathing, and activities as necessary.	
Gradually increase activity. Avoid increasing the pulse rate more than 30 beats above the resting heart rate.	An increase in heart rate of more than 30 beats above the resting heart rate indicates intolerance of activity and adversely affects oxygen supply and demand. With tachycardia, there is a reduction of diastolic filling time and oxygenation of the myocardium.

NURSING DIAGNOSIS: HIGH RISK FOR ALTERED NUTRITION: LESS THAN BODY REQUIREMENTS

Risk Factors
- Fatigue
- Pain
- Anorexia
- Antimicrobial therapy

Patient Outcomes
- The patient will demonstrate adequate nutritional intake and maintenance of positive nitrogen balance.
- Body weight will be stable.

Nursing Interventions	Rationales
Assess nutritional status, including weight, appetite, usual eating patterns, and intake of protein and calories.	Early identification of risk can result in more effective treatment.
Review serum prealbumin at regular intervals.	Prealbumin levels are sensitive indicators of malnutrition.
When oral intake is poor, conduct a calorie count for 3 days and collaborate with the dietitian to determine nutritional goals.	
Medicate for pain.	Pain frequently leads to anorexia.
Have dietary personnel plan menus that include individual food preferences.	

Nursing Interventions	Rationales
Collaborate with physicians regarding enteral nutrition or total parental nutrition (TPN) when unable to maintain adequate oral intake.	Enteral nutrition is preferable when the patient has a functioning GI tract because of the risk of sepsis associated with TPN.

NURSING DIAGNOSIS: KNOWLEDGE DEFICIT

Related To no prior experience with critical illness and complex medical regimen

Defining Characteristics
Verbalization indicating inadequate understanding of disease process and treatment regimen

Patient Outcomes
The patient will verbalize and demonstrate knowledge related to
- risk factors
- necessary precautions
- signs and symptoms of infective endocarditis
- the American Heart Association prophylaxis recommendations

Nursing Interventions	Rationales
Assess knowledge related to infective endocarditis.	The best method of endocarditis prevention is knowledge about the risks for developing the disease.
Review the information outlined in the Infective Endocarditis Teaching Plan (Table 8.1).	
Provide written instructions.	Learning occurs more readily when at least two teaching strategies are used.

DISCHARGE PLANNING/CONTINUITY OF CARE

- Patients are discharged from the hospital when afebrile with negative blood cultures.

- Discharge occurs before antimicrobial therapy is completed.
- Establish IV access through a peripheral or central line.
- Coordinate in-home or outpatient antimicrobial therapy with the discharge planner.
- Monitor laboratory work such as peak and trough antibiotic levels and BUN and creatinine levels.
- Facilitate physician follow-up.
- Assess need for household assistance.
- Coordinate in-home or outpatient physical therapy in the deconditioned elderly patient.

Table 8.1 • Infective Endocarditis Teaching Plan

The patient will:
1. Verbalize definition of infective endocarditis. Infective endocarditis is an infectious and inflammatory condition involving the heart valves and endothelial lining of the heart.
2. Verbalize risk factors for developing infective endocarditis:
   a. People who have one or more of the following are at risk:
      (1) Abnormal or damaged heart valves
      (2) Artificial heart valves
      (3) Congenital heart defects
      (4) Patch grafts used on or near the heart
   b. Specific life-style risks include IV drug abuse and acupuncture.
3. Verbalize self-care activities needed to help prevent or treat infective endocarditis:
   a. Notify all physicians and dentist of endocarditis risk before appointment or procedure is scheduled.
   b. Verbalize indications for prophylactic antibiotic therapy (see Table 8.2).
   c. Verbalize importance of dental hygiene:
      (1) Avoid gum trauma by brushing teeth regularly with a soft bristle toothbrush.
      (2) Avoid instruments that cause the gums to bleed, such as Waterpiks and toothpicks.
      (3) Have routine dental examinations.
      (4) Maintain properly fitted dentures to avoid oral ulcers.
   d. Verbalize signs and symptoms of infective endocarditis. The patient should report signs or symptoms: persistent fever, night sweats, chills, generalized fatigue, anorexia, abnormally painful joints, shortness of breath.
   e. Demonstrate ability to measure body temperature.
   f. Verbalize importance of carrying identification stating at risk for infective endocarditis:
      (1) Wallet cards
      (2) Medic alert jewelry

▼

Table 8.2 • American Heart Association Standard Regimen for Dental, Oral, or Upper Respiratory Tract Procedures

Amoxicillin	3.0 g orally 1 hr before the procedure and 1.5 g 6 hr after first dose

For patients allergic to penicillin:

Erythromycin	Erythromycin ethylsuccinate 800 mg, or erythromycin stearate, 1.0 g orally two hours before the procedure and 500 mg six hours after the first dose.
Clindamycin	300 mg orally one hour before the procedure and 150 mg six hours after the first dose.

Adapted from A. S. Dajani, A. L. Bisno, K. J. Chung, D. T. Durack, M. Fried, M. A. Gerber, A. W. Karchmer, H. D. Millard, S. Rahimtoola, S. T. Shulman, C. Walanakunakorn, & K. A. Taubert, (1992, March/April). Prevention of bacterial endocarditis. *Heart Disease and Stroke*, pp. 53–57.

REFERENCES

Dajani, A. S., Bisno, A. L., Chung, K. J., Durack, D. T., Fried, M., Gerber, M. A., Karchmer, A. W., Millard, H. D., Rahimtoola, S., Shulman, S. T., Walanakunakord, C., & Taubert, K. A. (1992, March/April). Prevention of bacterial endocarditis. *Heart Disease and Stroke*, pp. 53–57.

Scrima, D. A. (1987). Infective endocarditis: Nursing considerations. *Critical Care Nurse, 7*(2), 47–50, 52, 54–56.

Snelson, C., Cline, B. A., & Luby, C. (1993). Infective endocarditis: A challenging diagnosis. *Dimensions of Critical Care Nursing, 12*(1), 4–16.

Trausch, P. A. (1988). Infective endocarditis: Nursing care and prevention. *Progress in Cardiovascular Nursing, 3*(2), 45–53.

$\mathcal{H}$YPERTENSIVE CRISIS

Patricia A. Burke, RN, MS, CCRN

Hypertensive crisis is the name given to hypertensive emergencies severe enough to cause permanent end-organ damage. The myocardium, kidneys, and brain are at particular risk as blood pressure elevates to critical levels that cause arterial endothelial injury. Organ ischemia ensues from the resultant platelet aggregation, intravascular coagulation, arteriolar spasm, and leakage of fluids into perivascular tissues.

There is no single set of clinical findings that constitute a hypertensive emergency. The usually normotensive patient whose diastolic blood pressure suddenly exceeds 120 mmHg requires rapid treatment. So does any hypertensive patient who presents with one or more of the following: hypertensive encephalopathy, grade III or IV retinopathy (papilledema), acute myocardial infarction (MI), acute left ventricular failure, unstable angina, pulmonary edema, dissecting aortic aneurysm, cerebrovascular accident (CVA), head trauma, burns, postoperative bleeding, renal insufficiency, or eclampsia.

The goal of treatment in hypertensive crisis is to lower the blood pressure to a level that lessens the risk of neurological, renal, and/or myocardial damage without compromising central and peripheral tissue perfusion.

ETIOLOGIES

- Chronic moderate to severe essential hypertension
- Increased renin-angiotensin level (renin-secreting tumors, renal disease)
- Renovascular hypertension
- Acute glomerulonephritis
- Drug noncompliance or withdrawal resulting in rebound hypertension
- Pheochromocytoma
- Central nervous system injuries
- Burns
- Drug actions and side effects (oral contraceptives, tricyclics, amphetamines, sympathomimetics, steroids, nonsteroidal anti-inflammatory agents, ergot alkaloids, beta blockers in hypoglycemic patients

- Drug interactions [monoamine oxidase (MAO) inhibitors and tyramine, fentanyl-diazepam-oxygen combination]

CLINICAL MANIFESTATIONS

- Often asymptomatic until advanced or severe
- Lethargy
- Dizziness
- Blurred vision
- Temporary paralysis
- Altered mental status
- Headaches, usually in the morning
- Epistaxis
- Coma
- Chest pain (may be angina or dissecting aneurysm)
- Congestive heart failure
- Cardiac dysrhythmias
- Nausea
- Vomiting
- Seizures

CLINICAL/DIAGNOSTIC FINDINGS

- Any combination of clinical manifestations
- Elevated blood urea nitrogen (BUN) and serum creatinine
- Hematuria, red cell casts, proteinuria on urinalysis
- Renal bruits
- Retinal papilledema, hemorrhages, and exudates
- Left ventricular hypertrophy on ECG
- Ischemic changes on ECG
- Murmur of aortic insufficiency
- Rales
- S_3 gallop
- Pulmonary edema
- Depleted serum sodium with hypovolemia
- Hyperkalemia (if renal failure)

NURSING DIAGNOSIS: HIGH RISK FOR ALTERED TISSUE PERFUSION—CENTRAL AND PERIPHERAL

Risk Factors
- Damaged arteriolar intima
- Platelet aggregation and intravascular coagulation

- Altered cerebral autoregulation
- Rapid reduction in blood pressure

Patient Outcomes
- Mean arterial blood pressure (MAP) will be reduced by approximately 25% in 1 hr.
- Diastolic blood pressure will be reduced to 100–110 mmHg.
- Encephalopathy, aortic dissection, myocardial ischemia, acute renal insufficiency, and retinopathy will be prevented or detected early.

Nursing Interventions	Rationales
Assess cardiovascular status: blood pressure, heart rate, cardiac rhythm, peripheral perfusion, lung sounds, and subjective complaints.	Patients with hypertensive crisis risk aortic dissection, which may present as sudden, sharp chest or back pain. Myocardial ischemia is also observed and may manifest itself as anginal pain, left ventricular failure, dysrhythmias, poor peripheral perfusion, rales, and dyspnea.
Assess neurological status.	Confusion, decreased level of consciousness, sensorimotor deficits, nausea, vomiting, and seizures are all signs of hypertensive encephalopathy. If these signs are persistent, CVA and/or increasing intracranial pressure should be ruled out and sedatives withheld.
Assess patient's vision for gross visual changes. Check retinas with ophthalmoscope for hemorrhages, exudates, and blurring of the optic disk.	Presence of papilledema and retinal hemorrhages and exudates precede renal damage in severe hypertension and are reliable signs of malignant hypertension. Gross visual changes may indicate rising intracranial pressure.

Nursing Interventions	**Rationales**
Assess BUN, serum creatinine, urinalysis, and volume and quality of urine output.	When hypertension is severe and/or long-standing, progressive renal insufficiency occurs and will be reflected in rising BUN and serum creatinine. As nephrons are damaged, they hemolyze red cells, causing hematuria. The kidney's concentrating abilities are impaired. Proteinuria also ensues as the glomerulus becomes more permeable. Oliguria may be reflective of renal failure or decreased glomerular filtration rate (GFR) as blood pressure falls in the patient with long-standing hypertension. Acute end-organ changes require admission to the intensive care unit (ICU); patients without end-organ damage can have their blood pressures reduced gradually over 24–48 hr.
Administer antihypertensive medications as ordered, observing blood pressure closely during initial treatment (see Table 9.1 for commonly used drugs).	In the long-standing hypertensive patient, cerebral autoregulation is reset and is thus less sensitive to rapid changes in blood pressure. A sudden fall in blood pressure may cause cerebral ischemia, whose symptoms may include transient ischemic attacks (TIAs), CVA, blindness, seizures, loss of consciousness, or coma.

NURSING DIAGNOSIS: HIGH RISK FOR FLUID VOLUME DEFICIT SECONDARY TO SERUM SODIUM DEPLETION

Risk Factors
- Pressure-related diuresis
- Continued hypertension due to activation of vasopressor hormones

Patient Outcomes
Fluid volume status will return to normal, as evidenced by
- normal cardiac output and filling pressures
- normal sinus rhythm on ECG
- serum sodium between 136 and 145 mEq/L

Table 9.1 • Drugs Used to Treat Hypertensive Crises

Drug	Usual Dose/Route	Mechanism of Action	Side Effects
Sodium nitroprusside (Nipride, Nitropress)	0.5–10 µg/kg/min intravenous (IV)	Arteriolar and venous vasodilator; reduces cardiac preload and afterload without reflex tachycardia; immediate onset; lasts 3–5 min after discontinuance	Cyanide and thiocyanate toxicity, hypotension
IV nitroglycerin (Nitrobid IV, Nitrostat IV, Tridil)	5–100 µg/min IV	Dilates venous capacitance vessels; dilates arterioles in large doses; reduces mean arterial blood pressure without significantly affecting stroke volume or cardiac output; dilates coronary collateral vessels; immediate onset; metabolites (dinitrates and mononitrates) have half-life of 1–4 min	Hypotension. Sudden discontinuance can cause rebound cardiac ischemic symptoms such as angina.
Clonidine HCl (Catapres)	Initial dose 0.1–0.2 mg IV, then 0.05–0.1 mg orally every hour to maximum of 0.7 mg. Can be given concomitantly with nitroprusside; in such cases, it is given every 2 hr.	Decreases systemic vascular resistance, renal vascular resistance, heart rate, and blood pressure, while preserving glomerular filtration rate and postural reflexes	Dry mouth, orthostatic symptoms, constipation, sedation, vertigo
Diazoxide (Hyperstat)	1–2 mg/kg over 10–15 s, repeat at 10–15-min intervals IV; as an infusion, given undiluted at 15–30 mg/min	Arteriolar dilatation; no effect on venous capacitance; lowers blood pressure in 3–5 min, duration 2–4 hr after stopped	Hypotension, reflex tachycardia. Avoid use in the cardiac patient.

Table 9.1 • Continued

Drug	Usual Dose/Route	Mechanism of Action	Side Effects
Hydralazine (Apresoline)	0.1–0.5 mg/kg IV; maximum dose 25 mg	Arterial vasodilator; lowers blood pressure 10–80 min after infusion	Hypotension, reflex tachycardia. Avoid use in cardiac patient.
Verapamil (Isoptin, Calan)	3–25 mg/hr IV continuously	Decreases cardiac contractility, relaxes smooth muscle, slows cardiac conduction, and decreases heart rate	Decreases heart rate and conduction changes in patients with coronary artery disease, especially patients on digitalis or beta blockers
Nifedipine (Procardia)	0..25–0.5 mg/kg sublingually, or have alert patient bite the capsule, then swallow with water	Decreases cardiac contractility; relaxes smooth vascular muscle; slows heart rate; onset 10–15 min; duration 3–6 hr	Difficult to control decline in blood pressure; hypotension
Labetalol HCl (Normodyne, Trandate)	0.5–2 mg/min IV infusion, or miniboluses of 20–40 mg every 10–15 min	Arteriolar dilatation; decreased pulmonary vascular resistance; onset about 5 min, 3–6 hr duration of action	Hypotension; bronchospasm in asthma, chronic obstructive pulmonary disease; heart failure
Phentolamine (Regitine)	5 mg IV	Alpha-adrenergic effect, vasodilatation of vascular smooth muscle	Hypotension, tachycardia, cardiac dysrhythmias, weakness, dizziness, flushing, nausea, vomiting, nasal congestion
Captopril (Capoten)	6.25–25 mg PO	Inhibits angiotensin I–converting enzyme; suppresses renin-angiotensin-aldosterone system; lowers blood pressure in 15–30 min	Hypotension, particularly in patients who are on diuretics
Trimethaphan camsylate (Arfonad)	40–90 µg/kg/min continuous infusion or 1000 mg/L	Ganglionic blocker, vasodilation Onset of action 5–10 min; duration 5–10 min	Urinary retention, hypotension, paralytic ileus, paralysis of pupillary reflex, dry mouth

▼

Nursing Interventions	Rationales
Administer normal or hypertonic saline as ordered.	These solutions restore circulatory volume and sodium.
Assess blood pressure, central venous pressure (CVP), and pulmonary capillary wedge pressure as fluid volume is restored.	The predisposition of hypertensive patients to cardiovascular disease puts them at risk for fluid volume overloading. A rising resting heart rate during fluid replacement may be a sign of circulatory overload in the patient with cardiovascular disease.
Assess serum electrolytes during volume replacement.	Periodic electrolyte checks help guide the choice of intravenous fluids for volume replacement. An increase in ectopy may indicate hypokalemia, requiring potassium replacement.

NURSING DIAGNOSIS: KNOWLEDGE DEFICIT

Related To lack of previous exposure to hypertensive problems, denial, or anxiety

Defining Characteristics
Patient unable to relate pertinent information about prescribed antihypertensives.
Patient requests information about hypertension treatment.

Patient Outcomes
Patient will
- explain importance of hypertension treatment and consequences of foregoing such treatment
- verbalize signs and symptoms of poor control and/or complications and a mechanism of reporting them
- verbalize a plan for follow-up care

Nursing Interventions

Discuss with alert patient (and significant other, if possible) the ramifications of untreated hypertension. Discuss factors and behaviors that may predispose to hypertensive crises, such as antihypertensive noncompliance. Provide written instructions regarding signs, symptoms, home blood pressure monitoring, treatment, dietary considerations, recommended health behaviors, and resources for questions/follow-up. Involve home care and social services as necessary.

Rationales

Information, resources, and support do not absolutely guarantee adherence to medical regimens; however, without information, the best intentioned of patients cannot make informed decisions about their health behaviors.

DISCHARGE PLANNING/CONTINUITY OF CARE

- Ensure appropriate teaching regarding hypertension, including risks, aggravating factors, and treatment.
- Facilitate follow-up visit with physician.
- Attempt to link the patient without a physician to a primary care provider.

REFERENCES

DeAngelis, R. (1991). The cardiovascular system. In J. G. Alspach (Ed.), *Core curriculum for critical care nursing* (pp. 132–299). Philadelphia: Saunders.

Keller, K. B., & Lemberg, L. (1991). Hypertensive crisis. *Heart & Lung, 20,* 421–424.

O'Donnell, M. E. (1990). Assessment of the patient with malignant hypertension. *Dimensions of Critical Care Nursing, 9*(5), 280–286.

Smith, C. B., Flower, L. W., & Reinhardt, C. E. (1991). Control of hypertensive emergencies. *Postgraduate Medicine, 89*(5), 111–116, 119.

$\mathcal{C}$EREBRAL VASCULAR ACCIDENT

Sandra A. Kopczenski, RN, BSN

A cerebral vascular accident (CVA) is a syndrome that results from an interruption of the blood supply to a portion of the brain. Most commonly, a CVA results from occlusive disorders such as embolic occlusion of a cerebral blood vessel or thrombus formation in a cerebral artery. A CVA can also be hemorrhagic in origin, resulting from the rupture of a cerebral blood vessel.

ETIOLOGIES

- Thrombosis
  - atherosclerosis
  - inadequate cerebral perfusion
  - polycythemia
- Embolism
  - rheumatic heart disease
  - bacterial endocarditis
  - atrial fibrillation
  - myocardial infarction
  - valvular heart disease
  - congestive cardiomyopathy
  - fat emboli
  - air emboli
  - cardiac surgery
  - polycythemia
  - hypercoagulability
  - oral contraceptives
- Hemorrhage
  - malignant hypertension
  - brain tumor
  - ruptured arteriovenous malformation
  - trauma

136

- ruptured cerebral aneurysm
- bleeding disorders

CLINICAL MANIFESTATIONS

Neurological deficit, dependent on location and severity of the CVA:
- Alteration in level of consciousness (LOC)
  - confusion
  - lethargy
  - stupor
  - coma
  - seizure activity
- Motor deficit
  - hemiplegia
  - weakness
  - psychomotor disturbance
  - facial paralysis
  - balance disturbance
- Brain stem dysfunction
  - gaze deviation
  - ptosis
  - dysconjugate eye movement
  - diplopia
  - nystagmus
  - facial asymmetry
  - absence of gag reflex
  - tongue deviation
  - abnormal pupil size, shape, or reaction to light
  - bradycardia
  - increased systolic blood pressure
  - widened pulse pressure
  - abnormal respiratory rate or rhythm
  - altered thermoregulation
  - nausea and vomiting
  - dysrhythmias
- Sensory deficit
  - paresthesia of face, hand, or foot
  - hemiparesthesia
- Cognitive impairment
  - short attention span
  - dysphasia
  - aphasia
  - memory impairment
  - agnosia
  - apraxia
  - headache

CLINICAL/DIAGNOSTIC FINDINGS

Noninvasive tests
- Computerized axial tomography (CAT) scan
  - Differentiates hemorrhagic and occlusive CVA. Hemorrhagic CVA is immediately seen as a white lesion. Rules out tumor as the cause of neurological deficit.
- Magnetic resonance imaging (MRI)
  - Provides detailed information on the nature and extent of the CVA.
  - Detects necrotic tissue or ischemic tissue.
- Electroencephalogram (EEG)
  - Used to diagnose neurological dysfunction or seizure activity and monitor response to therapy.
- Electrocardiogram (ECG)
  - bradycardia
  - dysrhythmias
- Biochemical profile
  - Arterial blood gases: Respiratory acidosis (low pH and high $PaCO_2$) or respiratory alkalosis (high pH and low $PaCO_2$) coupled with hypoxemia may be the result of increased intracranial pressure.
  - Coagulation parameters: A decreased platelet count, decreased fibrinogen, increased prothrombin time (PT), or increased partial thromboplastin time (PTT) may indicate coagulopathy as the source of the CVA.
- Renal function tests
  - Elevated BUN and serum creatinine may indicate concomitant renal infarction.
- Blood cultures
  - Obtained in the presence of fever or known/suspected valvular disease.

Invasive tests
- Cerebral angiography
  - Detects vascular abnormality.
  - Cerebral blood flow studies
  - Can be used to verify brain death. Serially can detect changes in cerebral blood flow.
- Lumbar puncture
  - Grossly bloody spinal fluid indicates a cerebral hemorrhage has occurred. Lumbar puncture is also useful to rule out meningitis.

NURSING DIAGNOSIS: ALTERED TISSUE PERFUSION— CEREBRAL

Related To impaired cerebral circulation

Defining Characteristics
Alteration in level of consciousness

Motor deficit
Sensory deficit
Cognitive impairment
Headache
Brain stem dysfunction

Patient Outcomes

Patient will demonstrate neurological stability, as evidenced by
- stable level of consciousness
- halt of neurological deterioration
- improvement in neurological status
- stable respiratory rate and rhythm, blood pressure, and heart rate
- normal body temperature
- absence of dysrhythmias

Nursing Interventions	Rationales
Monitor neurological status by assessing LOC, verbal response, pupil shape and reactivity, motor response, ocular movement, facial symmetry, gag reflex, tongue position, extremity strength, temperature, heart rate and rhythm, respiratory rate and rhythm, and blood pressure.	Identification of the neurological deficit or neurological change will guide nursing intervention.
Evaluate the comatose patient by assessing response to noxious stimuli. If no response is noted, observe for response when nailbed pressure is applied bilaterally or central muscle group is stimulated. Observe for facial grimace, withdrawal from painful stimulus, or abnormal flexion or extension posturing:	
1. Assess gag reflex by directly stimulating the back of the throat. This should result in a gag response.	The gag reflex assesses function of cranial nerves 9 (glossopharyngeal) and 10 (vagus).
2. Assess corneal reflex by lightly touching the cornea with a wisp of cotton or gauze. This should result in a blink response.	The corneal reflex assesses function of cranial nerves 5 (trigeminal) and 7 (facial).

Nursing Interventions	**Rationales**
3. Assess doll's eyes (oculocephalic reflex) by turning the head briskly from side to side. Observe for eye movement. If doll's eyes are present, the eyes move in the opposite direction of the head. When doll's eyes are absent, eye gaze follows the direction of head movement.	Absent doll's eyes indicates brain stem dysfunction.
4. Assess cold calorics (oculovestibular reflex) by injecting ice water through a catheter placed into the patient's ear as ordered by the physician. An intact occulovestibular reflex results in lateral nystagmus with deviation of the eye toward the irrigated ear, then rapid movement away.	An abnormal response to cold calorics indicates brain stem dysfunction.
5. Assess Babinski reflex by stimulating the lateral aspect of the sole of the foot with constant pressure from the heal across the ball of the foot.	Dorsiflexion of the great toe and fanning of the other toes is considered an abnormal response indicating upper motor neuron dysfunction.
Institute appropriate pharmacological therapy, assess response and monitor for complications of drug use. (See Table 10.1 for action, response, and complications of specific drug herapy.)	
Maintain patent airway. Intubation should be accomplished in the presence of respiratory depression, decreased level of consciousness, or impaired cough or swallow reflexes.	Hypoxia or hypercapnia lead to vasodilation and increased ICP.
Hyperventilate using mechanical ventilation to achieve a $PaCO_2$ of 25–30.	Hyperventilation causes cerebral vasoconstriction and reduces intracranial pressure (ICP).

Nursing Interventions

Position patient optimally:

1. Elevate head of bed 20°–30°
2. Trendelenburg position should be avoided.
3. Maintain head and neck in a midline position.
4. Minimize conditions that increase intra-abdominal or intrathoracic pressure. Coughing, sneezing, the Valsalva maneuver, and positive end-expiratory pressure are examples.
5. Allow rest periods between nursing intervention.

6. Decrease environmental stimuli.

Aggressively treat hyperthermia by administering antipyretics as ordered and using cooling devices to maintain normal temperature.

Rationales

This enhances cerebral venous drainage.

This allows the ICP to return to baseline between nursing interventions.

Cerebral metabolic rate increases as body temperature increases.

NURSING DIAGNOSIS: IMPAIRED PHYSICAL MOBILITY

Related To neuromuscular impairment

Defining Characteristics
Inability to move within the environment
Expression of fear with movement
Impaired range of motion
Muscle weakness
Impaired coordination
Imposed restrictions of movement

Patient Outcomes
Patient will
- not experience any body system complications associated with immobility
- participate in a supervised physical rehabilitation program
- adjust to permanent mobility impairments

Table 10.1 • Pharmacological Therapy for Acute CVA

Drug	Response	Complication
Corticosteroids	The goal of steroid use is to reduce cerebral inflammation and decrease intracranial pressure (ICP). Routine steroid use in the brain-injured patient is controversial since documentation of effectiveness is limited.	Fluid retention, electrolyte imbalance, elevated blood glucose
Diuretics: mannitol, furosemide	Diuretics administered following a CVA decrease cerebral edema, resulting in a decreased total brain mass and decreased ICP. Expected responses to diuretic therapy include an increase in urine output, decrease in weight, decrease in ICP, halt of neurological deterioration, and improvement in neurological status. Mannitol is an osmotic diuretic. Cerebral fluid is mobilized into the vascular space within 15 min of administration. Furosemide is a loop diuretic that acts by inhibiting chloride transport. It can be given in conjunction with osmotic diuretics.	Fluid imbalance, electrolyte disturbance, hypotension, and metabolic alkalosis. ICP may increase after discontinuing osmotic diuretics such as mannitol. *Note*: Assess Mannitol solutions for crystals. If crystals are present, the solution should not be administered. If furosemide is given in conjunction with dilantin, dilantin absorption is decreased.
Barbiturates: thiopental, pentobarbitol	Barbiturates are cerebral vasoconstrictors that decrease cerebral blood volume and therefore decrease ICP. Barbiturates can also be used to induce coma and reduce cerebral metabolism. Barbiturates suppress seizure activity.	Neurological assessment parameters are limited during barbiturate administration. Serial computerized axial tomography scans may be necessary for ongoing patient assessment. Barbiturate administration may precipitate hypotension or respiratory depression.

Table 10.1 • Continued

Drug	Response	Complication
Anticoagulants: heparin	Anticoagulants reduce the risk of further cerebral infarction. Heparin inhibits clotting by inactivating thrombin. This prevents new clots from forming but does not lyse existing clots. The partial thromboplastin time should be maintained at 2–2$\frac{1}{2}$ times normal during heparin therapy.	Complications of anticoagulant administration include bleeding (hematuria, petechiae, blood in gastric secretions or stool, bleeding from puncture sites or wounds, bruising) and neurological deterioration. Anticoagulants should not be administered until hemorrhagic CVA has been ruled out.
Antihypertensives: Nitroprusside, hydralazine, labetalol	Antihypertensive agents are administered to reduce systolic blood pressure. Target blood pressure is based on the type of CVA and the patient's baseline blood pressure. Nitroprusside is a potent vasodilator. Hydralazine is an arterial vasodilator. Labetalol is a beta-adrenergic blocker.	Complications of antihypertensive administration include hypotension, headache, dizziness, bradycardia or tachycardia, and vomiting.

Nursing Interventions	Rationales
Monitor for complications of immobility by assessing skin condition, lung sounds, respiratory rate and rhythm, cough, gastrointestinal and genitourinary status, extremity strength, and movement. The most common complications include skin breakdown, infection, loss of muscle strength or mass, paralytic ileus, and constipation.	The sooner a complication is detected, the sooner it can be treated and permanent damage can be prevented or minimized.
Reposition every 2 hr.	This redistributes pressure and allows circulation to be restored to areas of pressure.

Nursing Interventions	Rationales
Give skin care to prominent areas or potential breakdown areas with every position change.	
Utilize pressure relief devices such as specialty bed mattress.	
Perform active/passive range-of-motion exercises.	Range-of-motion prevents muscle weakness or contractures.
Establish short-term activity goals in collaboration with patient and other disciplines. Focus on improvements in mobility and strength.	Achievement of realistic short-term goals encourages the patient toward further rehabilitative efforts.
Advance activity level as tolerated and assess tolerance.	
Encourage independence as appropriate.	
Maintain proper body alignment during activity and rest.	Proper body alignment prevents contractures and maintains pressure relief.
Administer stool softeners as necessary.	
Instruct in the following: 1. mobility regimen 2. ROM exercises 3. quad setting exercises 4. transfer technique 5. skin inspection	
Initiate consultation to physical therapy when physiologically stable.	
Initiate occupational therapy consult when physiologically stable.	

NURSING DIAGNOSIS: SELF-CARE DEFICIT

Related To neurological/musculoskeletal impairments

Defining Characteristics

Inability to eat, dress, engage in activities of daily living, or personal hygiene activities

Patient Outcomes

The patient will

- participate in self-care activities, including personal hygiene, eating, dressing, and activity
- effectively use adaptive devices

Nursing Interventions	Rationales
Monitor for effective swallowing of liquids and solids.	Swallowing should be carefully assessed, as aspiration pneumonia is a common complication of CVA.
Evaluate need for continuing care referrals on discharge.	
Evaluate need for adaptive grooming or eating devices.	
Establish short-term, attainable self-care goals in collaboration with patient, family, and other disciplines.	A clear team approach facilitates achievement of goals.
Establish daily routine in collaboration with the patient, encorporating therapies, self-care activities, diversional activities, and rest.	A planned routine balances activity and rest periods so the patient can benefit optimally from therapy.
Position optimally to enhance ability to eat or perform self-care tasks.	Helping the patient to be independent when possible decreases frustration and enhances self-esteem.
Position objects within the patient's visual fields.	Visual fields may be impaired.
Promote family involvement in self-care activities.	
Instruct patient on use of adaptive devices.	

NURSING DIAGNOSIS: IMPAIRED VERBAL COMMUNICATION

Related To cognitive impairments

Defining Characteristics

Unable to speak or speaks wih difficulty
Difficulty expressing self verbally
Inappropriate verbalization

Patient Outcomes

The patient will
- establish a means to communicate with caregivers and family members
- adapt to permanent communication barriers

Nursing Interventions	Rationales
Initiate consultation to speech therapy.	
Establish short-term, attainable communication goals in conjunction with the patient and speech therapist.	Achieving goals provides positive reinforcement to the patient.
Evaluate various methods of communication with the patient and family.	Use multiple methods of communication to supplement verbal communication.
Use nonverbal communication strategies.	Communication is facilitated through the use of gestures and nonverbal cues.
Avoid rushing the patient during attempts to speak.	Effective communication is less likely when the patient is stressed.
Encourage clear communication, implementing the following: 1. Speak to the patient directly and speak distinctly. 2. Speak slowly and use simple directions. 3. Do not raise voice volume unless the patient is hearing impaired.	The patient may have difficulty sorting essential from nonessential information.
Acknowledge the frustration associated with communication impairments. Reinforce successful communication.	Acknowledgment and understanding of feelings strengthen the nurse-patient relationship.
Provide support and reassurance to the patient and family.	Decreasing family stress allows the family to direct more energy toward assisting the patient.
Facilitate communication between the patient and family members.	
Explain cause of communication impairments to patient and family.	Increasing the family's understanding of the patient's problem increases their ability to reestablish communication.

Nursing Interventions	Rationales
Instruct family on effective communication strategies.	

DISCHARGE PLANNING/CONTINUITY OF CARE

- Provide ongoing reports to family, including status and prognosis.
- Anticipate transfer to rehabilitation or extended care facility if appropriate.
- Assess patient and family needs if discharge to home is appropriate.
- Initiate home care referrals.

REFERENCES

Leahy, N. (1990). Stroke: But which kind? *Emergency Medicine, 21*(14), 112–127.

Leahy, N. (1991). Complications in the acute stages of stroke: Nursing's pivotal role. *Nursing Clinics of North America, 26*(4), 971–984.

Phipps, M. (1991). Assessment of neurologic deficits in stroke: Acute-care and rehabilitation implications. *Nursing Clinics of North America, 26*(4), 957–970.

Romito, D. (1990). A critical path for CVA patients. *Rehabilitation Nursing, 15*(3), 153–156.

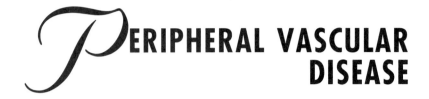

PERIPHERAL VASCULAR DISEASE

Lori A. Hislop, RN, BSN, CCRN

Peripheral vascular disease (PVD) is a disease of the arteries of the extremities which results in decreased flow of oxygenated blood to the tissues. Peripheral vascular disease refers to atherosclerosis outside of the heart. The most common presentation of PVD is that affecting the legs. However, it may also affect the renal arteries, abdominal aorta, carotid arteries, and brachial and subclavian vessels. With the exception of renal and carotid artery stenosis, claudication is often the presenting symptom. With renal artery stenosis, uncontrolled hypertension is often the first presenting symptom. Carotid artery stenosis usually presents as a transient ischemic attack (TIA) or cerebral vascular accident (CVA). However, it may be identified as an asymptomatic bruit on a routine exam.

Advances in medical therapies, balloon catheter technology, and surgical interventions have led to multiple treatment options for the patient with PVD. Antiplatelet and anticoagulant regimens, walking programs, and risk factor modification are just some of the medical therapies that may be offered. Catheter technology has led to the use of balloon angioplasty, stents, atherectomy, and lytic agents. Finally, new microsurgical techniques, dacron grafting, and advancement in anesthesia offer yet other approaches to treatment of the disease.

Early diagnosis and intervention of PVD has been shown to improve mortality and morbidity. Peripheral vascular disease is often misinterpreted as arthritic conditions, muscle strains, or back problems. With a national focus on healthy and active lifestyles we are seeing more physically active adults who present with claudication symptoms at a seemingly younger age. That coupled with an increased public awareness of the disease and its symptoms may lead to an earlier diagnosis.

Whether acute or chronic, PVD constitutes a threat to the involved limb. The factors influencing mortality and morbidity include prompt recognition, protection of the limb from all trauma and early, restoration of blood flow. (Table 11.1)

Table 11.1 • Treatment Options in PVD

Interventional Approaches

Percutaneous transluminal angioplasty (PTA)	Inflation of a balloon-tipped catheter across a lesion (plaque). This opens the lumen and restores blood flow to the distal extremity.
Atherectomy	Directional (shaving) or rotational (high-speed burr) atherectomy removes plaque. The devices may be useful in heavily calcified lesions, total or subtotal occlusion and long lesions.
Laser	A special type of light wave which can be controlled to carry energy in the form of heat. The laser waves are confined in an angioplasty catheter with the tip of the catheter being made of metal that heats when the laser is turned on. The laser catheter tip is placed across the lesion, the laser energy is turned on, and the subsequent heat production vaporizes the obstruction.
Lytic therapy	Prolonged infusion of lytic agent at the site of narrowing to dissolve existing thrombus prior to angioplasty.
Stent	A stainless steel mesh coil that acts as a scaffolding device to give support to the artery and maintain patency. The stent is deployed to the site using an angioplasty catheter. Stent trials are currently being conducted at limited test centers. Some have already been approved for use. Stents may be placed in the superficial femoral artery, iliac artery, distal abdominal aorta, renal artery, and subclavian artery.

Surgical Approaches

Bypass	Surgical rerouting of blood flow around an obstruction. Surgical bypass may be done with reversed vein or Dacron grafting in the lower extremities, renal artery, or subclavian artery. Intraoperative transluminal balloon dilatation may be used as a combined procedure at the time of surgery.
Endarterectomy	Surgical removal of atheromatous plaque. This may be performed in any artery as a direct method of revascularization, more commonly used in the carotid artery. May also be used in combination with surgical bypass.

Medical Approaches

Risk factor modification	Reduce or eliminate risk factors to slow the progression of disease.
Walking program	Walk up to 2–3 miles per day to build up collateral circulation. This approach is most beneficial in the mild to moderate stages of PVD.
Drug therapy	Aspirin, dypridamole, warfarin sodium, pentoxifylline. See Table 11.3.

▼

ETIOLOGIES

- Peripheral vascular disease: Risk factors include: smoking, male gender, advancing age, family history of PVD, history of preexisting vascular disease (i.e., coronary artery disease), obesity, diabetes

mellitus, sedentary lifestyle, hypertension, hypercholesterolemia, and hypertriglyceridemia.
- Restenosis of a previous angioplasty site: a healing process involving deposition of smooth-muscle cells and fibroblasts at an angioplasty site. When this reparative process is excessive, it may encroach on the lumen of the artery.
- Anastomotic site narrowing in a previously placed bypass graft (i.e., femoral-femoral bypass, femoral-popliteal bypass)
- Progression of peripheral vascular disease in existing bypass or native vessels
- Acute arterial occlusion: thrombosis, arteriosclerosis obliterans, myeloproliferative disease, arterial trauma, fibromuscular dysplasia, arterial spasm
- Chronic arterial occlusion: arteriosclerosis obliterans, arteritis (connective tissue disease, Takayasu's disease), congenital arterial narrowing

CLINICAL MANIFESTATIONS

Lower extremities
- Intermittent claudication
- Coolness of the extremity
- Pallor
- Hair loss at the distal extremity
- Rest pain
- Non-healing wounds or ulcers
- Dry skin and nail beds
- Diminished pulses
- Parasthesias
- Paralysis (acute occlusion)
- Male impotence (seen in iliac artery stenosis)

Upper extremities
- Intermittent claudication or arm fatigue (i.e., after brushing hair, holding arm up above the level of heart, repetitive movements)
- Coolness of the extremity
- Pallor
- Diminished pulses
- Parasthesias
- Paralysis (acute occlusion)
- Blood pressure in the affected arm lower (or undetected) as compared to unaffected arm

Renal artery stenosis
- Uncontrolled hypertension (refractory to medical management and/or a reduction in risk factors) often with a recent onset and diagnosis
- Renal insufficiency (elevated creatinine, elevated blood urea nitrogen)
- Possible auscultation of bruit over renal artery

- Atrophy of affected kidney [diagnosed by ultrasound, computerized tomography (CT) scan, or angiography]

Carotid artery stenosis
- Possible auscultation bruit over the affected artery
- History of transient ischemic attacks/stroke

CLINICAL/DIAGNOSTIC FINDINGS

Non-invasive studies
- History and physical
- Electrocardiogram (ECG)
  - The ECG may be within normal limits.
  - Assess the ECG for changes of previous myocardial injury or patterns of ischemia (ST- and T-wave changes). This is important to evaluate since up to 50% of patients presenting with PVD may have significant obstructive coronary artery disease (CAD).
  - ECG abnormalities may include ST-segment depression, ST-segment elevation (hyperacute), T-wave inversion, decreased R-wave height, intraventricular or bundle branch block conduction disturbances, and dysrythmias (usually ventricular extrasystoles).
- Ankle/brachial index, a ratio of the systolic pressure at the ankle divided by the brachial systolic pressure:
  - normal ≥ 0.95
  - mild to moderate arterial insufficiency = 0.50–0.70
  - severe arterial insufficiency < 0.50
- Ultrasound/color flow Dopplers, a noninvasive measurement of blood flow that allows for the prediction of the degree of stenosis and the level at which it occurs
- Peripheral treadmill test, a noninvasive, objective measurement of claudication symptoms. The treadmill is placed at a 10% grade and the patient is asked to walk at 2 miles per hour until symptoms of claudication appear. Time is measured at the first onset of pain and the patient is asked to continue until he or she is unable to continue. The time is recorded at the termination of the exam. The patient is allowed to recover and the length of time for recovery from pain is also recorded.
- Laboratory studies
  - Lipid profile: Note elevation of cholesterol, triglycerides, and low-density lipoprotein (LDL). High-density lipoprotein (HDL) normal or low.
  - Complete blood count: Assess for undiagnosed anemia, which may contribute to claudication symptoms.
  - Electrolytes: Assess for hypokalemia, which may provoke ventricular extrasystoles.
  - Creatinine/blood urea nitrogen: Assess for elevation of values that indicate preexisting renal insufficiency, which may require further investigation.

- Liver function studies: Assess for elevation of values which may point toward chronic liver congestion secondary to right-sided heart failure or may be consistent with primary liver dysfunction. Values may be elevated following chronic exposure to toxic substances such as alcohol and drugs, particularly lipid-lowering agents. The cause of abnormalities must be investigated as most primary medications are cleared through the liver.
- Stool for occult blood: A positive stool specimen should be investigated as to the source of occult loss. This is especially important if the patient needs to be placed on antiplatelet or anticoagulation therapy and/or if anemia is diagnosed.

Invasive Studies
- Angiography: Injection of contrast dye into the circulation. Diagnostic and imaging equipment produces detailed images of the arterial blood flow and direction of the flow. Abnormal findings consist of stenoses in the vessel, evidence of dissection or "dye staining" outside the vessel, or aneurysmal dilatation. The expected blood flow is antegrade. However, with critical lesions in the cerebral system in particular, retrograde blood flow may be seen in the vetebral arteries.

NURSING DIAGNOSIS: HIGH RISK FOR ACUTE PAIN

Risk Factors
- Tissue hypoxia/ischemia
- Muscle tension/spasm
- Parasthesias

Patient Outcomes
The patient verbalizes that the pain is relieved or adequately controlled.

Nursing Interventions	Rationales
Assess the level of discomfort using established pain assessment tools and rating scales.	A baseline assessment is key to evaluating response to therapy.
Identify and avoid pain-aggravating factors, such as	Items that constrict may contribute to ischemia by compressing arterial flow or precipitating edema (poor venous return) and thereby increase pain.

Nursing Interventions	Rationales
1. tight shoes, stockings, or dressings	
2. extremes of temperature	
3. weight of bed linens on extremity	
4. infrequent use of pain medication or pain medication poorly absorbed	
5. too much activity	Activity such as walking and stair climbing may contribute to ischemia and claudication by increasing the demand for oxygen in the tissues.
Identify and promote pain-relieving interventions, including:	
1. Avoid tight clothing, shoes, and dressings.	
2. Use a bed cradle to keep the linens off of the extremity.	
3. Use lukewarm water for bathing.	Temperature extremes risk the chance of burns. Parathesias prevent sensations of harmful temperature extremes.
4. Teach the patient to hold the extremity below the level of the heart.	This promotes dependent circulation and may help relieve severe rest pain.
5. Limit activity. Encourage frequent rest periods.	This decreases oxygen demand.
Medicate with prescribed analgesia.	Ischemic pain is often complex and difficult to control.
Offer pain medications at regular intervals.	Keeping a constant level of analgesia may avoid severe bouts of pain. Pain control may be achieved by altering the route of administration or use of combined therapies such as nonsteroidal antiinflammatory agents with narcotic agents.

Nursing Interventions	Rationales
Evaluate the effectiveness of the pain control regimen.	The present regimen may be inadequate if the patient's pain has changed from the initial assessment.
Consider alternative measures to control pain, that is, patient-controlled analgesia (PCA), epidural analgesia, and narcotic and non-narcotic combination therapy.	Pain may be derived from several origins such as sympathetic, inflammatory, and ischemic. Pain intervention should focus on the source of the pain.
Consider adjunctive methods for pain management, for example, 1. massage 2. relaxation techniques 3. warm or cool compresses 4. repositioning	The current prescribed pain regimen may be more effective if combined with relaxation and other techniques. Alternative methods of pain management may decrease oxygen demand, relax muscles in spasm, and improve oxygen supply to tissues by dilating the arterial bed.
Consult with the physician if pain control is ineffective to consider an alternative regimen and/or consider consulting an anesthesiologist for further recommendations.	Pain is complex and may have several origins. An anesthesiologist may contribute expertise in the area of pain management.

NURSING DIAGNOSIS: HIGH RISK FOR IMPAIRED SKIN INTEGRITY

Risk Factors
- Decreased circulation
- Parasthesias

Patient Outcomes
The patient will maintain baseline level or improved skin integrity, as evidenced by absence of or no further skin breakdown.

Nursing Interventions	Rationales
Inspect lower extremities and document findings.	A baseline assessment is necessary to evaluate therapy.

Nursing Interventions	Rationales
Inspect feet daily and record findings.	Prospective identification of skin disruption is important to prevent complications of PVD. Ongoing evaluation of status is the basis for determining whether prevention is effective.
Protect skin integrity by 1. use of foot cradle 2. use of heal protectors 3. application of lambswool or dry gauze 2 × 2 between toes 4. avoidance of tape on lower extremities	Use of preventative devices may decrease the potential for skin breakdown by decreasing pressure, preventing maceration of tissues (by keeping dry), and preventing trauma.
Teach patient and family how to perform routine daily foot inspections and proper foot care: 1. Lower extremities should be inspected daily. A mirror can be used to see the bottom of feet. 2. Family member should perform inspection if patient's vision is poor or mobility is limited. 3. Proper fitting shoes should be worn. 4. Shoes should be inspected before putting on each time: hand placed inside shoe to feel for foreign objects or irregular surfaces which may injure the foot. 5. Feet should be kept clean and dry. 6. Toenails should be routinely trimmed (every 30–60 days).	 Detection of new ulcers, cuts, or trauma will increase the opportunity for early treatment, healing, and minimal complications. Tight shoes may contribute to ischemia, while loose fitting shoes may produce blisters or trauma. The hand may be able to detect rough surfaces that may go undetected by the foot affected by parasthesias. Some insurance companies will provide coverage for a podiatrist to provide this service every 30–61 days.

Nursing Interventions	Rationales
7. Crossing legs should be avoided at all times.	Crossing legs may contribute to edema by decreasing venous return. Significant edema may produce secondary constriction of the arterial bed and compound ischemia.
8. Shoes should be worn at all times when walking.	Shoes may prevent trauma from such things as a stubbed toe or stepping on objects.
9. Cream should be applied to dry areas of feet.	Dry skin may crack and become a source of infection
10. Patient should be routinely followed by a physician and/or podiatrist.	Follow-up care is essential because of the progressive nature of the disease.
Teach patient and family about the effect of chronic ischemia precipitating parasthesias. Instruct the patient to report the onset of parasthesia to his or her physician. Encourage safety precautions to prevent injury such as: 1. Remove obstructive furniture that may cause injury. 2. Avoid throw rugs, which may slip or create loss of balance. 3. Test bath water with hand or use a thermometer if the hands are also affected. Hot water may burn a foot with parasthesia.	Chronic ischemia may result in damaged or impaired peripheral nerves. To meet the metabolic needs, the arterioles of the muscles will steal from the arterioles supplying the peripheral bed.

NURSING DIAGNOSIS: HIGH RISK FOR INJURY

Risk Factors
- Invasive arterial procedure (i.e., angiogram, angioplasty, or surgery)
- Severe arterial peripheral vascular disease

Patient Outcomes
- The patient will maintain adequate tissue perfusion (equivalent or improved from the baseline assessment).

- Alterations in vascular supply will be promptly recognized.
- Body temperature will remain below 100 °F.
- The vascular access site will remain clean, dry, and intact without erythema, drainage, or increased echymosis from the baseline assessment.
- The patient will maintain perfusion, motion, and sensation of the extremity that is unchanged or improved from the baseline assessment.

Nursing Interventions	Rationales
Assess dorsalis pedis and posterior tibial pulses on admission, before procedures, immediately postintervention and then every 15 min for 1 hr, every 30 min for 4 hr, and every 2–4 hr and prn.	Frequent checks following procedures will assist in recognizing changes and allow for prompt intervention. The use of a Doppler may be necessary when pulses are weak.
Assess pulse, motion and sensation of *both* extremities with each vital sign check.	The risk of distal embolization to *either* lower extremity is present if angioplasty catheters pass into the abdominal aorta or iliac arteries by a brachial, ipsilateral, or contralateral femoral approach. A sudden change in assessment may indicate acute arterial occlusion.
Monitor vital signs, including temperature, every 4 hr and prn. Report fever above 100 °F.	A new fever may signal infection. Blood pressure and pulse may decrease with vasovagal reaction. Blood pressure may decrease following renal artery angioplasty. The renin-angiotensin system is interrupted when the renal artery blood flow is reestablished.
Monitor hemoglobin, hematocrit, and white blood cell count.	A decrease in hemoglobin and hematocrit may indicate bleeding. An elevated white blood cell count may signal infection.
Inspect access site and note evidence of oozing, hematoma formation, or tenderness.	Early detection may minimize complications.
Assess ankle/brachial index on admission and 24 hr postprocedure and prn. To perform; calculate the systolic ankle pressure divided by the systolic brachial blood pressure.	Measuring the ankle/brachial index will give an *objective* value to lower extremity pulses and will assist in detecting changes in the arterial pressure to the extremity.

Nursing Interventions	Rationales
Maintain bedrest (post–sheath removal) for: 1. 8 hr—femoral approach 2. 3 hr—brachial approach	
Following removal of arterial sheaths, apply direct manual pressure for 20 min and then apply a dressing to the site for 12–24 hr.	This will obtain hemostasis at the site and minimize the potential for bleeding. Direct manual pressure is preferred so that hemostasis is adequately obtained. Avoid a vascular clamp during the first 20 min of compression, as this is likely to be the time a patient may experience a vasovagal reaction and should be directly observed.
Following sheath removal, postpercutaneous transluminal angioplasty (PTA) consider application of a 5–10-lb sandbag or vascular clamp to the access site after hemostasis is obtained, especially if the patient is anticoagulated for the procedure. Note: Avoid if the angioplasty site is in the iliac artery or proximal superficial femoral artery and the femoral access site is ipsilateral. This may contribute to slow blood flow over the angioplasty site and create the potential for thrombus and acute closure of the lumen.	Additional and prolonged compression at the site (at a pressure less than the patient's systolic pressure) will allow flow to the affected extremity but also promote platelet aggregation to form a plug at the access site. This can also prevent pseudoaneurysm or hematoma formation by decreasing the potential for a false lumen or internal bleeding.
Avoid elevation of the head of the bed greater than 15°–30° for the first 8 hr following femoral sheath removal.	Bending at the groin site may create pressure and cause rebleeding to occur. In obese patients and those with pendulous abdomens, bending will obscure direct vision and access to the site in the event of bleeding or hematoma formation.

Nursing Interventions	Rationales
Avoid constriction to the affected extremity (i.e., restraints, tight socks or shoes).	Constrictive devices may contribute to ischemia and decrease arterial blood flow. Socks or shoes may make it difficult to accurately and quickly assess pulse, motions, sensation, and color of extremity.
Maintain a dressing over the access site for 24–72 hr following sheath removal. Use a pressure dressing (gauze and tape) or transparent dressing. Promptly change any saturated dressing. Do not hesitate to remove all dressings at any time if the dressings obscure the ability to adequately assess the access site.	A dressing over the site will minimize the risk for bacterial invasion of the site with subsequent infection. A gauze dressing offers the advantage of better absorption of drainage, adds additional pressure to the site, and also reminds the patient not to bend the affected site. Transparent dressings allow direct visualization of the site at all times and create an occlusive barrier to prevent infection. Transparent dressings are often more comfortable and create less risk of tape trauma or skin reaction to tape.
Mark hematoma size (use a skin marker) every hour and prn.	
Measure access site girth every hr and prn.	An increase in girth may signal hematoma formation without signs of obvious external bleeding.
Auscultate for bruits over the access site each shift.	A bruit may indicate pseudoaneurysm formation.
Report deterioration or absence of pulse or sudden pain in the extremity immediately to the physician.	These signs indicate severely compromised arterial circulation. Early institution of treatment will minimize complications.

NURSING DIAGNOSIS: HIGH RISK FOR FLUID VOLUME EXCESS

Risk Factors
- Contrast dye load during angiogram, angioplasty, or intraoperative angiograms
- Preexisting renal insufficiency
- Preexisting left ventricular dysfunction

Patient Outcomes
- Electrolytes, creatinine, and blood urea nitrogen (BUN) will remain unchanged from the baseline assessment or will return to baseline at the time of discharge (2–4 days).
- Urine output exceeding 30 mL/hr or 720 mL per 24 hr will be maintained.
- Weight will remain unchanged from the baseline or return to baseline at the time of discharge.

Nursing Interventions	Rationales
Assess and report signs and symptoms of fluid overload (i.e., dyspnea, rales, peripheral edema, or jugular venous distention) to the physician.	Contrast dye may precipitate acute tubular necrosis and transient renal failure leading to fluid volume excess and congestive heart failure.
Monitor laboratory values and report elevation in BUN, creatinine, and potassium.	Baseline values are necessary to follow the trend during the hospital course.
Alert the physician if the creatinine is above 1.3 mg/dL or if the patient is diabetic to consider intravenous hydration before the procedure.	Diabetes predisposes to renovascular disease and therefore a decreased ability to clear the contrast agents. Prehydration may assist in clearance of the contrast.
Administer intravenous fluids as prescribed.	Hydration will assist in clearance of the contrast agent. In the setting of preexisting renal insufficiency consideration may be given to hydration with intravenous fluids for 8–10 hr preprocedure.

Nursing Interventions	Rationales
Administer osmotic diuretics as prescribed.	Osmotic diuretics (i.e., mannitol 10%) may increase the osmotic pressure of glomerular filtration, inhibit tubular reabsorption of water and electrolytes, and elevate blood plasma osmolality resulting in enhanced flow of water into extracellular fluid. This increases circulating volume, promotes renal perfusion pressure and subsequently promotes diuresis. This promotes rapid clearance of the contrast agent and therefore limits the necrosing effect on the kidney tubule.
Encourage oral intake of fluids for the first 24 hr following the procedure.	Hydration is essential to assist in renal clearance of the contrast agent used.
Record hourly urine output if catheterized.	
Record 24 hr intake and output during the hospital course.	
Report urine outputs below 30 mL/hr or below 720 mL in 24 hr.	A decrease in urine output may indicate decreased renal function. This may be related to the ability to clear the contrast or may be prerenal in origin (i.e., decreased perfusion from low cardiac output or dehydration). Correlate with laboratory values.
Weigh daily and report weight gain of 2 lb in 24 hr or 5 lb in 48 hr to physician. Consider fluid restriction.	Rapid weight gain with renal insufficiency predisposes to congestive heart failure, especially if preexisting left ventricular dysfunction is present.

NURSING DIAGNOSIS: HIGH RISK FOR ALTERED TISSUE PERFUSION—CEREBRAL

Risk Factors
- Invasive vascular procedure (angiogram, angioplasty, or surgery)
- vascular insufficiency

Patient Outcomes
Baseline level of consciousness will be maintained, as evidenced by
- alert, oriented mental status
- ability to communicate
- ability to move all extremities
- ability to appropriately sense and respond to noxious stimuli
- ability to swallow

Nursing Interventions	Rationales
Assess neurological status for baseline evaluation and then with each vital sign check and prn. Complete an assessment following any surgical or interventional procedure.	Chronic arterial insufficiency places the patient at risk for TIAs or potentially a stroke. Ruptured plaque or clot may break free and embolize into a segment of the cerebral arterial bed, resulting in a stroke. Similarly, patients may experience TIA or stroke during cerebral angiography. The contrast temporarily displaces oxygenated blood. This may precipitate a neurological event in an already compromised patient.
Assess the following: 1. orientation (person, place, time) 2. motor strength (hand grasp, dorsiflexion: toes and heels) 3. pupil reaction 4. ability to follow commands and act appropriately 5. ability to swallow food and fluids without coughing, drooling, or pooling food in mouth	

Nursing Interventions	**Rationales**
Report changes in neurological status promptly to the physician.	Early intervention may minimize complications. If the event is precipitated by a drop in blood pressure, for example, prompt fluid resuscitation or administration of inotropes may restore cerebral perfusion. Administration of anticoagulants may redue the chance of recurrent strokes if embolic in nature.

NURSING DIAGNOSIS: KNOWLEDGE DEFICIT

Related To complex treatment plan

Defining Characteristics

Verbalizations indicating inadequate understanding, misinterpretation of information, or misconception of desired health behavior
Lack of recall of information given
Inability to follow instructions

Patient Outcomes

The patient and family will
- verbalize understanding of peripheral vascular disease, including
  - etiology
  - personal risk factors
  - treatment options (see Table 11.1):
- verbalize understanding of procedures (i.e., angiogram, interventional therapies, surgery, medical treatment)
- comply with postprocedure follow-up and care
- notify staff immediately of any symptom or problem
- verbalize knowledge of routine foot care and follow-up care

Nursing Interventions	**Rationales**
Assess the patient's level of education and understanding	A baseline level of understanding is necessary to build teaching strategies.
Present information from a standardized teaching plan for PVD and document teaching done (see Table 11.2).	

Nursing Interventions	Rationales
Review investigational procedures and permits verbally and provide written information. Review surgical procedures and expected outcomes. Allow adequate time for reading and reviewing materials.	
Encourage questions and verbalization of concerns and fears. Ask open-ended questions and allow adequate time to discuss concerns.	
Teach signs and symptoms of coronary vascular insufficiency.	Coexistent CAD may be present and must be suspected. As many as 50% of patients with PVD have CAD.
Explain the importance of reporting subjective symptoms (i.e., acute leg or foot pain, coolness, numbness of the extremity). Emphasize that time is critical when dealing with complications.	The patient may fear further procedures or limb loss or may deny symptoms.
Begin discharge teaching and planning. Include 1. risk factor modification 2. follow-up protocols and procedures 3. restenosis versus progression of disease 4. medications (see Table 11.3)	

DISCHARGE PLANNING/CONTINUITY OF CARE

- Review patient learning needs regarding PVD. Assess knowledge level, correct misconceptions, and reinforce information.
- Include spouse, family members, and significant others in discharge teaching.
- Prepare a road map of medications, dosages, and dose schedule. Ensure that the patient is sent home with necessary prescriptions.
- Assess need for community resources and provide with appropriate referrals.
- Consult a dietitian to meet with patient and spouse/significant other to review recommended dietary guidelines.

- Review patient's risk factors for PVD. Ask the patient to list and develop strategies to modify his or her lifestyle.
- Discuss warning signs or possible complications that require immediate attentions:
  - sudden onset of leg pain/pain in affected extremity
  - sudden onset of a change in temperature in an extremity
  - new wound or ulcer on leg or foot
  - onset of drainage, redness, or separation of surgical incision line
  - fever > 100.5 °F, especially that occurring after surgical intervention
  - onset of numbness, tingling, or burning in the extremity, especially at rest
  - pain in an extremity that keeps patient awake at night (rest pain)
  - sudden change in skin color: blanched, hyperemic, black necrotic areas
  - sudden swelling of extremity
- Review mechanisms to access health care system in the event of complications:
  - Call 911 or emergency response team for sudden or severe problems.
  - Contact the physician for new changes that are not severely limiting but may be compromising the ability to perform activities of daily living.
- Discuss signs and symptoms of CAD (i.e., fatigue, chest pain, shortness of breath, decreased activity tolerance). Reinforce that as many as 50% of patients with PVD may also have some degree of CAD.
- Provide written schedule for follow-up appointments, examinations, and tests.
- Provide written foot care instructions that include
  - outline of daily foot care routine (washing, inspection, nail clipping, etc.)
  - recommended exercise and daily activities
  - safety guidelines (i.e., wearing shoes at all times when up walking, purchasing well-fitting shoes, and breaking them in gradually)

Table 11.2 • Teaching Plan for the Patient With PVD

The patient will be able to:
- Define risk factors for peripheral vascular disease.
- Identify his or her risk factors for PVD.
- Prioritize his or her risk factors and identify specific lifestyle modifying behaviors.
- Define what claudication is and what causes it.
- Discuss the signs and symptoms of peripheral vascular disease:
  - Claudication (upper extremity versus lower extremity)
  - Physical signs of chronic limb ischemia (i.e., hair loss, nonhealing wound)
  - Uncontrolled hypertension
  - Transient ischemic attack/stroke
- Discuss treatment options for PVD (see Table 11.1):
  - Interventional approaches
  - Surgical approaches
  - Medical management
- Discuss the purpose of treatment options for PVD. Understand the progressive nature of the disease and the potential complications, including limb loss.
- List pharmacological agents prescribed for the patient, their mechanism of action, and the desired effect. See Table 11.3.

Table 11.3 • Pharmacological Agents Commonly Used in PVD

Aspirin	Impedes clotting by blocking prostaglandin synthesis, preventing formation of the platelet aggregating substance thromboxane A_2. Commonly used long term in patients with PVD and those who undergo interventional and surgical therapy.
Dipyridamole	Inhibits platelet adhesion and also inhibits the enzymes adenosine deaminase and phosphodiesterase. The value of dipyridamole remains controversial. However, it is an effective alternative for patients who are sensitive/allergic to aspirin. It may also be of benefit in the patient who is felt to be at too high of a risk to use warfarin sodium. It is frequently used following stent placement in combination with aspirin and warfarin sodium (triple therapy). Dipyridamole also exerts a vasodilating effect.

Table 11.3 • Continued

Warfarin sodium	Inhibits vitamin K–dependent activation of clotting factors II, VII, IX, and X which are formed in the liver. It is frequently used short term (sometimes long term) following successful lytic therapy, following stent placement, or if there is angiographic evidence of ulcerated plaque at the time of angioplasty. Following surgical endarterectomy, subendothelial layers may be exposed and become a highly thrombogenic surface. Warfarin sodium may be used short term (2–6 months) at which time endothelialization has occurred and the risk of acute thrombosis is minimized.
Pentoxifylline	Improves capillary blood flow by increasing erythrocyte flexibility and lowering blood viscosity. Its use is also controversial in that collateral blood flow and/or microcirculation must be present in order to benefit from the drug. This is a very useful agent in the early stages of PVD. In combination with risk factor modification and a stringent walking program, pentoxifylline can minimize claudication symptoms, thereby improving compliance with the exercise regimen.

REFERENCES

Bright, L. D., & Georgi, S. (1992). Peripheral vascular disease: Is it arterial or venous? *American Journal of Nursing, 92*(9), 34–43.

Creamer-Bauer, C., & Webber, M. (1990). Patient teaching strategies for peripheral laser procedures. *Progress in Cardiovascular Nursing, 5*(2), 50–58.

Ernst, E. E. W., & Matria, A. (1988). Exercise for intermittent claudication. *Cardiology Board Review, 5*, 82.

Fellows, E., & Jocz, A. M. (1991). Getting the upper hand on lower extremity disease. *Nursing 91, 21*(8), 34–42.

O'Brien, C. & Recker, D. (1992). How to remove a femoral sheath. *American Journal of Nursing, 92*(10), 34–37.

Payne, J. S. (1992). Alternatives for revascularization: Peripheral atherectomy devices. *Journal of Vascular Nursing, 10*(1), 2–8.

▼

Surgical Cardiovascular Problems and Interventions

▼

CARDIAC SURGERY: ACUTE PERIOPERATIVE PERIOD

Claire C. Elsesser, RN, BSN, CCRN

Cardiac surgery is performed to decrease symptoms and improve the quality of life of patients with heart disease. The technique of open heart surgery requires the use of cardiopulmonary bypass. This plan of care applies to any adult undergoing cardiac surgery.

ETIOLOGIES

- Coronary artery disease
- Valvular heart disease
- Congenital defects
- Ventricular aneurysm
- Cardiac tumor
- Pericardial disease
- Dysrhythmia management
- Cardiac trauma

CLINICAL MANIFESTATIONS (POSTOPERATIVE)

- Decreased cardiac output
- Dysrhythmias
- Left and/or right ventricular failure
- Bleeding
- Hypertension
- Hypoxia
- Hypothermia initially, possible low-grade fever
- Pain
- Decreased lung expansion

CLINICAL/DIAGNOSTIC FINDINGS (POSTOPERATIVE)

- Electrocardiogram (ECG) monitoring
  – bradycardia

- tachycardia
- premature atrial contractions
- atrial fibrillation or atrial flutter
- premature ventricular contractions
- ventricular tachycardia or fibrillation
- Twelve-lead ECG changes indicative of ischemia or infarction
- Hemodynamic monitoring
  - arterial blood pressure (ABP): hypotension, hypertension, labile
  - right atrial pressure (RAP): decreased in hypovolemia or increased in hypervolemia, ventricular failure, or cardiac tamponade
  - left atrial pressure (LAP): decreased in hypovolemia or increased in hypervolemia, left ventricular failure, or cardiac tamponade
  - pulmonary artery systolic (PAS) and diastolic (PAD) pressures: decreased in hypovolemia or increased in pulmonary hypertension, pulmonary disease, hypoxia, pulmonary emboli, or left ventricular failure
  - pulmonary capillary wedge pressure (PCWP): decreased in hypovolemia or increased in hypervolemia, left ventricular failure, or cardiac tamponade
- Thermodilution cardiac output decreased
- Mixed venous oxygen saturation (SvO_2) decreased
- Pulse oximetry: decreased oxygen saturation
- Chest x-ray: atelectasis, pulmonary infiltrates, interstitial edema, hemothorax, pneumothorax, widened mediastinum, abnormal intravenous line placement
- Laboratory
  - arterial blood gases (ABGs), electrolytes, complete blood count (CBC), creatinine, blood urea nitrogen (BUN), coagulation studies, cardiac enzymes, glucose, and chemistry profile: routine monitoring assists in detection of common postoperative conditions and complications

NURSING DIAGNOSIS: DECREASED CARDIAC OUTPUT

Related To decreased preload, increased afterload, dysrhythmias, and/or depressed myocardial contractility

Defining Characteristics
Unstable heart rate/rhythm and hemodynamic pressures
Hypothermia
Postoperative bleeding
Cardiac tamponade
Left and/or right ventricular failure
Compromised perfusion to body systems
Fatigue
Compromised wound healing

Patient Outcomes

Patient will

- maintain adequate perfusion of all body systems, as evidenced by cardiac output (CO) $\geq$ 4 L/min and cardiac index (CI) $\geq$ 2.5 L/min/m^2.
- maintain adequate preload, as evidenced by diastolic filling pressures returning to baseline (RAP 8–12 mmHg, PCWP/LAP 10–15 mmHg).
- maintain normal afterload status, as evidenced by ABP or mean arterial pressure (MAP) within prescribed parameters, systemic vascular resistance (SVR) 800–1200 dyn/s/cm^{-5}, and pulmonary vascular resistance (PVR) 37–250 dyn/s/cm^{-5}.
- maintain optimal heart rate (60–100 bpm) and rhythm.
- respond to pharmacological and mechanical support in the presence of decreased myocardial contractility.

Nursing Interventions	Rationales
Monitor and report early signs of decreased perfusion to body systems (decreased CO/CI, ABP, RAP, PCWP/LAP, SvO$_2$, urine output; tachycardia; cool, pale, and moist skin; decreased consciousness).	Decreased perfusion may cause multiorgan compromise.
Evaluate trends in hemodynamic pressures (ABP, PCWP/LAP, RAP).	Pressures fluctuate due to hypovolemia, bleeding, volume shifting, and body temperature changes.
Evaluate thermodilution CO and derived hemodynamic profile data.	A hemodynamic profile provides specific information about preload (PCWP/LAP, RAP), afterload (SVR, PVR), and contractility (left and right ventricular stroke work index, stroke volume index) status.
Monitor heart rate and rhythm: 1. Initiate antidysrhythmic therapy and/or pacing as indicated. 2. Monitor and replace serum potassium prn. 3. Use atrial electrograms to diagnose dysrhythmias prn. Note: Atrial electrograms, obtained via atrial epicardial wires, are useful to differentiate supraventricular from ventricular dysrhythmias.	Heart rate and rhythm must be optimized to maintain adequate CO.

Nursing Interventions	Rationales
Assess for signs of perioperative myocardial infarction: ECG changes, multilead ST-segment monitoring, 12-lead ECG, cardiac enzymes, chest pain, and signs of ventricular failure.	
Monitor trends in SvO_2	Continuous SvO_2 monitoring provides an indicator of the balance between oxygen supply and demand. Decreased SvO_2 relates to a decrease in CO, hemoglobin, and arterial oxygen saturation and/or an increase in oxygen consumption.
Assess core body temperature: 1. Apply heating blanket to bed prior to admission. 2. Institute rewarming measures on admission. 3. Minimize heat loss by covering patient and wrapping blanket around head. 4. Detect shivering and treat promptly. 5. Discontinue warming when temperature nears 37 °C.	Hypothermia is induced during cardiac surgery to protect the myocardium and reduce metabolic and oxygen demands. Slow rewarming is optimal (1 °C/hr). Shivering increases metabolic rate and myocardial work and may increase oxygen consumption by 400–500%.
Assess skin color, temperature, presence of edema, quality of peripheral pulses, and capillary refill time.	Patients with decreased CO will have poor perfusion indicated by cool, pale, mottled, and moist extremities, decreased quality of peripheral pulses, and capillary refill time under 3 s.
Evaluate hourly urine output, daily intake and output, and daily weight.	Status of fluid balance gives direction to plan of care.
Assess for evidence of bleeding: hourly chest tube drainage, incisional sites, chest x-ray, hematocrit and coagulation studies.	

Nursing Interventions	Rationales
Assess for signs of cardiac tamponade: decreased ABP, increased PCWP/RAP, widened mediastinum on chest x-ray, and sudden decrease in chest tube drainage. Prepare for emergency sternotomy at bedside and return to surgery.	Tamponade requires prompt surgical intervention to allow ventricular filling and contraction.
Report bleeding to surgeon and institute the following: 1. maintenance of chest tube patency [set prescribed level of suction and gently milk tube(s) to prevent clotting] 2. replacement with blood products as prescribed 3. preparation for possible return to surgery	
Replace volume as prescribed [e.g., autotransfusion or other blood transfusions, albumin, intravenous (IV) fluids] and monitor response.	Volume replacement augments CO by increasing preload. Fluctuations in preload status are common in the immediate postoperative period.
Titrate inotropic and vasoactive support medications for desired effects (e.g., dopamine, dobutamine, nitroprusside, nitroglycerin).	Inotropic infusions (dobutamine, dopamine) and vasoactive infusions (nitroprusside, nitroglycerin) are frequently used in combination to increase cardiac contractility and decrease afterload.
Monitor effectiveness of intra-aortic balloon pump (IABP) therapy if indicated.	This therapy decreases afterload and increases coronary artery and systemic perfusion.
Progress activity as tolerated (e.g., turn, elevate head of bed, dangle, chair, ambulate) and monitor response.	Activity is necessary to diminish postoperative complications, but the activity plan must be individualized.
Evaluate surgical incisions for adequate wound healing.	Decreased CO can compromise tissue oxygenation and wound healing.
Implement comfort strategies, such as pain medication, position changes, and relaxation techniques, to reduce pain and anxiety.	Pain and anxiety may contribute to increased afterload.

Nursing Interventions	Rationales
Involve patient and family in the plan of care: 1. provide focused information about condition and environment. 2. offer reassurance. 3. promote family visitation.	
Establish a plan to facilitate a smooth transition from the critical care unit.	Communication will provide for continuity of care and effective monitoring of individual problems, and may reduce fear or anxiety associated with transfer.

NURSING DIAGNOSIS: HIGH RISK FOR IMPAIRED GAS EXCHANGE

Risk Factors
- Anesthesia
- Atelectasis
- Cardiopulmonary bypass
- Decreased cardiac reserve
- Diaphragm dysfunction secondary to phrenic nerve injury
- History of lung disease
- Neurological compromise
- Pain
- Secretions
-

Patient Outcomes
Patient will
- maintain adequate gas exchange, as evidenced by ABGs within patient's normal range, clear breath sounds, clearing chest x-ray, and extubation within 24 hr.
- demonstrate an effective respiratory pattern, as evidenced by easy respirations, respiratory rate 15–25/min, and bilateral chest expansion.

Nursing Interventions	Rationales
Assess respiratory pattern, lung sounds, skin color, and changes in sensorium and report signs of respiratory compromise (labored breathing, tachypnea, adventitious breath sounds).	Early detection and prompt intervention may diminish complications.
Evaluate serial chest x-rays for status of lung fields and placement of endotracheal (ET) tube.	
Evaluate ABGs in conjunction with pulse oximetry and/or capnography (noninvasive end tidal CO_2 concentration) monitoring as indicated.	Pulse oximetry and/or capnography monitoring, combined with a respiratory assessment, may reduce the number of costly ABG draws used to evaluate gas exchange.
Monitor trends in SvO_2 when available.	Continuous SvO_2 monitoring provides an indicator of the balance between oxygen supply and demand.
Maintain airway patency: 1. Suction as indicated by lung auscultation. 2. Assess consistency and quality of secretions. 3. Maintain adequate humidification. 4. Detect and respond to signs of airway obstruction: thick secretions, increasing airway pressure on ventilator gauge, and signs of respiratory compromise.	Airway obstruction is a potential complication. It may occur more frequently in ventilator-dependent patients, despite adequate airway patency measures.

Nursing Interventions	**Rationales**
Increase or decrease ventilation and oxygenation to maintain ABGs: 1. Establish synchrony with ventilator. 2. Evaluate response to positive end-expiratory pressure (PEEP). 3. Assess readiness to wean and initiate weaning plan in consideration of risk factors. 4. Elicit patient support during weaning by providing reassurance and instruction on the use of controlled breathing or relaxation techniques. 5. Assess quality of spontaneous respirations and intervene for signs of weaning intolerance. 6. Consult with physician regarding placement of tracheostomy tube in ventilator-dependent patient.	Mechanical ventilation is required in the acute postoperative period. Positive end-expiratory pressure may cause a decrease in CO, especially when the patient is hypovolemic. Success of weaning is based on multiple factors.
Promote lung expansion and secretion removal by implementing the following: 1. Elevate head of bed. 2. Reposition as tolerated. 3. Progress activity as tolerated. 4. Assist in performing thoracic exercises. 5. Establish an activity/rest schedule.	
Initiate postextubation pulmonary measures: oxygen and humidity therapy, cough and deep breathing exercises, incentive spirometry, and other respiratory treatments.	Preventive measures reduce the likelihood of pulmonary complications.
Manage pain.	Pain control will enhance the effectiveness of respiratory patterns and tolerance to respiratory therapies.
Provide adequate nutrition.	Energy stores must be maintained to sustain the work of breathing in a difficult to wean patient.

NURSING DIAGNOSIS: ACUTE PAIN

Related To cardiac surgery

Defining Characteristics
Verbalization of pain
Increased heart rate, blood pressure, respirations
Diminished respiratory excursion
Restricted activity
Muscle tension
Restlessness
Moaning
Nonverbal expression of pain
Diaphoresis

Patient Outcomes
Patient will
- verbalize relief of pain.
- identify strategies that promote pain relief.
- be able to rest.

Nursing Interventions	Rationales
Assess type of pain. Rate intensity of pain using a numerical (0–10) pain intensity scale.	It is necessary to differentiate surgical pain from angina. The pain experience can be better measured when objective tools are used.
Administer pain medication, monitor response, and evaluate effectiveness of the medication.	Morphine sulfate is routinely used in frequent small doses to manage acute postoperative pain. Hypotension may occur.
Encourage request of pain medication. Reassure patient and family that pain medication is necessary after surgery, and that pain will diminish over time.	
Medicate prior to activity, respiratory therapy, and painful procedures.	
Provide comfort measures: position changes, back rubs, and mouth care. During activity, splint chest incision using a folded blanket or firm pillow.	

Nursing Interventions

Involve patient and family in pain management plan:

1. Promote family visits and involvement in providing comfort measures.
2. Identify diversional activities.
3. Implement relaxation techniques when appropriate.

Rationales

NURSING DIAGNOSIS: HIGH RISK FOR ALTERED TISSUE PERFUSION—CEREBRAL

Risk Factors
- Altered sleep/rest patterns
- Cardiopulmonary bypass
- Cerebral ischemia
- Critical care environment
- Metabolic alterations

Patient Outcomes

Patient will
- be free of neurological impairment, as evidenced by return to preoperative level of consciousness, mentation, and motor and sensory function.
- be free from injury.

Nursing Interventions

Assess neurological status as patient emerges from anesthesia and continue to monitor for signs of neurological compromise. Assess level of consciousness, eye signs, movement, and sensation.

Rationales

Neurological compromise may range from mild confusion to transient or permanent deficits. A perioperative cerebrovascular accident (CVA) may result from prolonged periods of hypotension, emboli, or hemorrhage secondary to the anticoagulation used during cardiopulmonary bypass. The risk of cholesterol emboli is present with atherosclerotic cardiac disease, and calcium emboli may occur with valve disease.

Nursing Interventions	Rationales
Detect signs of confusion, anxiety, and/or hallucinations. Minimize environmental stimuli and promote rest. Use medications to manage symptoms as needed.	Postcardiotomy delirium may cause a variety of behavioral manifestations following cardiac surgery.
Assess vision.	Temporary or permanent loss of vision has been associated with occipital cortical infarcts in cardiac surgery patients.
Assess for peripheral neurological deficits.	Brachial plexus injury or ulnar nerve injury may result from nerve compression.
Maintain blood pressure to provide adequate cerebral perfusion.	
Utilize strategies to maintain orientation: eye glasses, hearing aid, clock, calendar, radio, windows, day/night routines, and family visits.	
Provide for safety: side rails, restraints prn, the family at bedside, and proper positioning.	

NURSING DIAGNOSIS: HIGH RISK FOR INFECTION

Risk Factors
- Surgical incisions
- Invasive lines, tubes, and devices
- Decreased cardiac output
- Intensive care environment
- Advanced age
- Impaired nutrition

Patient Outcomes
Patient will
- be free of infection, as evidenced by temperature within normal limits, white blood cell count normal, incision and invasive line sites clean and dry, lungs clear on auscultation, and cultures negative.
- experience normal wound healing.

Nursing Interventions	**Rationales**
Assess and report temperature elevation and other systemic and local signs and symptoms of infection. Culture any suspicious drainage.	Low-grade fever is a normal response to cardiac surgery, but always evaluate for the presence of infection. Common sites of infection include the lungs, urinary tract, incisions, and invasive line sites.
Assess for normal wound healing.	
Wash hands meticulously. Apply principles of aseptic technique in all nursing care.	
Leave incisional dressings in place for 24 hr; then provide incisional care per unit protocol.	
Follow protocol for invasive line care.	
Follow protocol for daily heart wire care.	
Discontinue invasive lines and tubes as soon as condition allows. Keep a written record of line insertion dates and change site of invasive lines according to protocol.	
Protect sternal incision from secretions during airway suctioning.	
Assist in coughing and deep breathing, engage in optimal respiratory treatments, and progress activity.	This enhances removal of secretions and reduces the risk of respiratory infection.
Administer antibiotics, antipyretics, and hypothermia therapy as prescribed.	

▼

DISCHARGE PLANNING/CONTINUITY OF CARE

- Prepare patient and family for transfer from the critical care unit. Discuss concerns and fears related to transfer.
- Facilitate a smooth transition of the patient and family from the critical care unit by documenting an individualized plan of care. Involve disciplines other than nursing as needed (e.g., social worker, chaplain).
- Assess readiness to learn and initiate a postoperative teaching plan with the patient and family.

REFERENCES

Gregersen, R. A., & McGregor, M. S. (1989). Cardiac surgery. In S. L. Underhill, S. L. Woods, E. S. Sivarajan Froelicher, & C. J. Halpenny (Eds.), *Cardiac nursing* 2nd ed., (pp. 537–560). Philadelphia: Lippincott.

Guzzetta, C. E., & Dossey, B. M. (1992). *Cardiovascular nursing: Holistic practice*. St. Louis, MO: Mosby Year Book.

Moorehouse, M. F., Geissler, A. C., & Doenges, M. E. (1987). *Critical care plans: Guidelines for patient care*. Philadelphia: Davis.

Neeley, J. M., Craft, M. S., & Branyon, M. (1991). Surgical management of coronary heart disease. In M. R. Kinney, D. R. Packa, K. G. Andreoli, & D. P. Zipes (Eds.), *Comprehensive cardiac care* (pp. 425–446). St. Louis, MO: Mosby Year Book.

Seifert, P. C. (1987). Surgery for acquired valvular heart disease. *Journal of Cardiovascular Nursing, 1*(3), 26–40.

Ward, C. R., & Monsein, S. (1990). The patient undergoing cardiac surgery. In M. D. Welsh & J. M. Clochesy (Eds.), *Case studies in cardiovascular critical care nursing* (pp. 231–267). Rockville, MD: Aspen.

Weiland, A. P., & Walker, W. E. (1986). Physiologic principles and clinical sequelae of cardiopulmonary bypass. *Heart & Lung, 15*, 34–39.

*C*ARDIAC SURGERY: RECOVERY PERIOD

Dona L. Hutson, RN, BSN

Coronary artery bypass grafting (CABG) involves connecting a new conduit for blood flow from the aorta or internal mammary artery (IMA) to the coronary artery distal to the site of stenosis. This results in improved circulation to the myocardium and improved myocardial oxygen supply. Coronary artery bypass grafting is a treatment, not a cure, for the underlying atherosclerotic process. However, this procedure has been shown to relieve ischemia and produce an improvement in symptoms and quality of life in select patient populations.

During the surgery, a median sternotomy is performed and the pericardium is opened. The IMAs are taken down from the chest wall and saphenous veins are harvested from the lower extremities. The patient is placed on cardiopulmonary bypass (CPB), which circulates and oxygenates the blood and allows for a motionless surgical field. Myocardial protection is achieved using continuous cross-clamping of the aorta and cardioplegia solutions. The bypass grafts are fashioned and anastomosed to the coronary arteries. Chest tubes are placed in the mediastinum and/or pleural spaces. Epicardial heart wires may be sewn to the anterior wall of the right ventricle and right atria and brought out via the skin over the left and/or right epigastrium. After adequate rewarming, the patient is weaned from CPB and heparin is reversed with protamine. After hemostasis is achieved, the incisions are closed using wire to the sternum and sutures to the fascia and skin.

ETIOLOGIES (INDICATIONS)

- Significant stenosis in one or more coronary arteries, that is, left main, left anterior descending, circumflex, and right coronary artery, resulting in myocardial ischemia
- Urgent/emergency situations: acute myocardial infarction (AMI), cardiogenic shock, unstable angina

- Failed or complicated percutaneous transluminal coronary angioplasty (PTCA): coronary dissection, acute closure of coronary artery
- Sudden hemodynamic compromise related to ischemia because of mechanical defects: papillary muscle rupture, ventricular septal defect (VSD), left ventricular aneurysm (LVA)
- Acute MI with recurrent angina despite maximum therapeutic intervention

CLINICAL MANIFESTATIONS (PREOPERATIVE)

- Angina pectoris
- Myocardial infarction (MI)
- Anxiety/apprehension
- Hypertension/hypotension
- Peripheral cyanosis
- Dysrhythmias
- Diaphoresis

NOTE: Refer to page 187 for postoperative clinical manifestations.

CLINICAL/DIAGNOSTIC FINDINGS (PREOPERATIVE)

- Biochemistry panel
  - lipid panel: hypercholesterolemia/hyperlipidemia
  - total cholesterol: high risk ≥ 240 mg/dL
  - low-density lipoprotein (LDL): high risk > 160 mg/dL
  - high-density lipoprotein (HDL): high risk < 35 mg/dL
  - triglycerides: high risk > 500 mg/dL
- Electrocardiography
  - acute changes: ischemia/AMI
  - tachycardia/bradycardia
  - artrial and/or ventricular ectopy
  - atrial or ventricular enlargement
- Echocardiography
  - wall thickness or wall motion abnormalities
  - atrial, septal or ventricular hypertrophy
  - decrease in left ventricular or right ventricular ejection fraction (LVEF/RVEF)
  - post-MI valvular insufficiency: ruptured mitral valve, papillary muscle dysfunction
  - post-MI aneurysm or clot formation
- Chest x-ray (CXR)
  - cardiomegaly
  - presence of congestive heart failure

- Exercise testing
  - subjective symptoms of ischemia
  - ST depression 1–2 mm
  - exercise hypotension
  - dysrhythmias
- Radionuclide imaging techniques
  - reversible defects indicating ischemia
  - fixed defects indicating severe ischemia or scar
- Right-sided heart catheterization
  - detection of acquired and/or congenital heart or pulmonary disease
  - increased pulmonary artery pressure and pulmonary artery wedge pressure
  - decreased RVEF
- Left ventricular catheterization/angiography
  - detection of stenoses of left main, left anterior descending, circumflex, or right coronary artery
  - hypokinesis or akinesis of left ventricle
  - decreased LVEF
  - detection of aortic or mitral valve abnormalities

NOTE: Refer to page 191 for postoperative clinical/diagnostic findings.

Valve repair or replacement

Valvular disorders are conditions resulting in abnormalities of the cardiac valve(s) and/or supporting structures. Treatment of valvular disorders consists of medical management of heart failure and subsequent multisystem pathophysiology and surgical intervention to repair or replace diseased valves. Valve rings are generally used to correct mitral or tricuspid valve insufficiency by restoring the valve annulus to a more normal size. During valve repair, a prosthetic ring is sewn in with felt buttress sutures and the chordae or leaflets of the valve may be repaired. Valve replacements are categorized as biological or mechanical. The biological types include bovine (Ionescu-Shiley), porcine (Carpentier-Edwards, Hancock), and homografts (cardaver aortic valve). The mechanical types include caged ball (Starr-Edwards), tilting disc (Bjork-Shiley, Medtronic-Hall) and bileaflet (St. Jude). In valve replacement, much of the diseased valve is removed. Sutures are placed in the valve annulus and through the sewing ring on the replacement valve. The valve is then seated, and the sutures are tightened. Postoperatively, continuous anticoagulant therapy is required for patients with mechanical valves and/or patients with atrial fibrillation to minimize the risk of thromboembolism.

ETIOLOGIES

- Infection or inflammatory process
  - infective endocarditis
  - rheumatic heart disease
  - acute rheumatic fever
  - myocarditis

- Congenital malformation
  - bicuspid aortic valve
  - mitral valve prolapse
  - ventricular septal defect
  - pulmonic stenosis
- Trauma
  - blunt force leading to rupture of chordae tendinae
- Ischemic damage
  - coronary artery disease (CAD) and left ventricular (LV) dilatation leading to displaced papillary muscles
  - rupture or fibrosis of papillary muscle
- Degenerative changes
  - systemic lupus erythematosus
  - myxomatous degeneration of the valvular leaflets
- Connective tissue disorder
  - Marfan's syndrome
- Calcific valvular disorder
  - calcification of aortic (most common) and mitral valve
  - annulus in the elderly

CLINICAL MANIFESTATIONS/DIAGNOSTIC FINDINGS (PREOPERATIVE)

Refer to Tables 13.1 and Table 13.2.

CLINICAL MANIFESTATIONS (POSTOPERATIVE/CABG AND VALVE REPAIR OR REPLACEMENT)

The patient may exhibit a number of abnormal clinical manifestations affecting many body systems:
- Cardiac
  - dysrhythmias, atrial, ventricular, heart block
  - palpitations
  - distant or muffled heart sounds
  - increased or decreased central venous pressure (CVP)
  - hypotension/hypertension
  - decreased peripheral pulses
  - pericardial friction rub
  - pulses paradoxus
  - neck vein distension
  - cool or moist skin
- Respiratory
  - increased respiratory rate
  - dyspnea
  - cyanosis
  - crackles, wheezes
  - increased capillary refill time (CRT)
  - restless state

Table 13.1 • Left-Sided Valvular Disorders

Name	Clinical Manifestations	Auscultation	Electrocardiogram	Chest X-ray	Echocardiogram
Mitral stenosis	Dyspnea, fatigue, palpitations; RV failure: hepatomegaly, splenomegaly, JVD, peripheral edema, hemoptysis, hoarseness, thromboembolism	Low-pitched, diastolic, rumbling murmur	Normal QRS, broad, notched P wave in lead II, atrial fibrillation, resting tachycardia	LA enlargement, prominent PA, enlarged right ventricle	LA enlargement, abnormal movement and thickening of valve leaflets and mitral valve orifice
Mitral regurgitation	Dyspnea: exertional, orthopnea, PND; fatigue, palpitations, crackles, JVD, embolization signs/symptoms of decreased CO and overtime; weakness, exhaustion, weight loss, cardiac cachexia	Systolic murmur, split S_2	Normal or LA enlargement, atrial fibrillation, LVH	Increased cardiac shadow, enlargement of left atrium and left ventricle; if acute, pulmonary congestion and pulmonary edema	Thickening of valve, valve prolapse, calcification of annulus, severity of regurgitant flow, dilated left atrium
Mitral valve prolapse	Slender physical build, mild to severe pain mimicking angina but unresponsive to rest or nitrates, variable symptoms: syncope, dyspnea, palpitations, anxiety, lightheadedness, tingling of hands, circumoral numbness	Midsystolic click, late systolic murmur	ST depression, premature atrial contractions, supraventricular tachycardia, premature ventricular contractions	Scoliosis, kyphosis, pectus excavatum	Abnormal billowing movement of the posterior leaflet, mitral regurgitation

Aortic stenosis (supravalvular, valvular, subaortic)	Chest pain associated with exertion, relieved with rest, syncope associated with orthostatic changes, orthopnea, crackles, later in disease process: marked fatigue, debilitated condition, angina	Aortic ejection murmur heard best at aortic region, S₄, systolic thrill, abnormal peripheral pulsations	LVH, atrial fibrillation, first-degree AV block, left bundle branch block	LA enlargement, pulmonary congestion	Leaflet thickening and decreased movement of the leaflets, calcification, dilated left ventricle, decreased LVEF, decreased aortic orifice with high-pressure gradient between left ventricle and aorta
Aortic insufficiency	Acute: volume overload on left ventricle, dyspnea, orthopnea, hepatomegaly, JVD peripheral edema, decreased diastolic blood pressure. Chronic: dyspnea, orthopnea, PND, fatigue	Blowing, diastolic high-pitched murmur, waterhammer peripheral pulses	LVH, may have prolonged PR interval	pulmonary congestion, heart failure	Ventricular volume overload (LVH), increased chamber size, aortic regurgitation

Note: RV = right ventricular, JVD = jugular venous distention, LA = left atrial, PA = pulmonary artery, PND = paroxysmal nocturnal dyspnea, CO = cardiac output, LV = left ventricular, LVH = left ventricular hypertrophy, AV = atrioventricular, LVEF = left ventricular ejection fraction, ECG = electrocardiogram, CXR = chest x-ray, ECHO = echocardiogram.

Table 13.2 • Right-Sided Valvular Disorders

Name	Clinical Manifestations	Auscultation	Electrocardiogram	Chest X-ray	Echocardiogram
Tricuspid stenosis	Easy fatigue, hepatomegaly cirrhosis, jaundice, malnutrition, peripheral edema, JVD; late sign: ascites	Diastolic rumble murmur heard best at the left sternal border, increased by inspiration	Small RSR[1] wave, lengthened PR; atrial fibrillation	RA enlargement	Thickened tricuspid valve leaflet, elevated RA pressure
Tricuspid insufficiency	Dyspnea, fatigue, right-sided heart failure: hepatomegaly, JVD, peripheral edema	Pansystolic murmur which increases in inspiration and decreases on expiration or Valsalva	Atrial fibrillation, RA or RV enlargement	RA or RV enlargement	Abnormal leaflet mobility, increased chamber size of RA and RV, valve incompetence
Pulmonic stenosis	Dyspnea, fatigue, systolic thrill	Harsh systolic murmur, split S_2	Normal to atrial fibrillation; V_1–V_6 abnormalities	Poststenotic dilation of pulmonary artery	Thickened valve leaflets
Pulmonic insufficiency	Dyspnea, fatigue, right heart failure: hepatomegaly, abdominal pain, ascites	Moderately pitched diastolic murmur	Normal to atrial fibrillation	RA or RV enlargement	Thickened valve leaflets with valve incompetence; pulmonary hypertension.

Note: JVD = jugular venous distention, RA = right atrial, RV = right ventricular.

- Renal
  - weight gain/edema
  - decreased urine output
- Hematological
  - sanguinous/serosanguinous incisional drainage
  - sanguinous/serosanguinous chest tube drainage
- Neurological
  - confusion and disorientation
  - focal deficits and paralysis
  - unequal pupils and reaction time
  - visual and memory deficits
- Gastrointestinal
  - nausea and vomiting
  - hypo- or hyperactive bowel sounds
  - abdominal distension
  - increased nasogastric suction drainage
- Pain
  - pain with or without movement
  - pain with inspiration

CLINICAL/DIAGNOSTIC FINDINGS (POSTOPERATIVE/CABG AND VALVE REPAIR OR REPLACEMENT)

- Cardiac
  - electrocardiogram (ECG): acute changes, surgical pericarditis
  - abnormal signal average ECG
  - echocardiogram (ECHO): abnormal wall motion, reduced contractility, pericardial fluid
  - multigated blood pool imaging scan (MUGA): abnormal LVEF/RVEF
- Respiratory
  - decreased tidal volume
  - arterial blood gases (ABGs): decreased PaO_2, elevated $PaCO_2$
  - CXR: hypoventilation, pneumothorax, atelectasis, pleural effusion
  - ventilation/perfusion scan: pleural fluid or findings consistent with pulmonary emboli
- Renal
  - elevated blood urea nitrogen (BUN)/creatinine
  - hypo- or hyperkalemia
  - hypomagnesemia
  - decreased or increased colloid osmotic pressure
- Hematological
  - decreased hemoglobin/hematocrit
  - decreased platelet count
  - increased prothrombin/partial thromboplastin (PT/PTT) time
  - coagulation panel: factor deficiencies
  - elevated white blood cell (WBC) count

- Neurological
  - abnormal computerized axial tomography of head
  - abnormal electroencephalogram
  - abnormal transcranial Doppler testing

NURSING DIAGNOSIS: ANXIETY

Related To need for surgery and uncertain outcome

Defining Characteristics
Facial tension
Hyperventilation
Crying
Trembling
Inability to concentrate
Emotional outbursts

Patient Outcomes
Patient and family will
- demonstrate a decrease in anxiety verbally and behaviorally.
- demonstrate/verbalize understanding of surgery including reason for surgery and expected outcome.
- demonstrate knowledge of pre- and postoperative care.
- verbalize concerns or fears related to surgery.

Nursing Interventions	Rationales
Assess patient/family members' current level of knowledge regarding cardiac surgery.	Use this as a guide to where teaching needs to be focused.
Assess patient/family members' current level of anxiety.	Reinforce that this is a stressful time for patients and family.
Reinforce the physician's explanation of surgery and reason why it is indicated, speaking slowly and calmly.	Anxiety may prevent understanding of physician explanations, and a review of this information is often necessary.
Explain preoperative testing or procedures as indicated.	Knowing what to expect will usually decrease the level of anxiety.
Provide written preopertive teaching information.	This information may answer many questions quickly, and family members may review it as needed.

Nursing Interventions	**Rationales**
Allow time for the patient/family to attend class or see preoperative teaching videotapes if they appear receptive to group teaching, or do individual teaching which includes the topics listed in Table 13.3.	
Utilize other interventions to decrease anxiety: 1. Explore feelings through open-ended questions: "What are you feeling? What are your questions?" 2. Teach simple relaxation techniques. 3. Encourage discussion of past and current methods of coping. 4. Offer antianxiety medication as prescribed.	In addition to standard teaching, many need individualized counseling to help them cope. Usual coping methods may be overwhelming by the stress of surgery, and specific intervention plus sedation may be indicated.

NURSING DIAGNOSIS: HIGH RISK FOR INFECTION

Risk Factors
- Surgical incisions
- Invasive lines, tubes
- Hospital environment
- Advanced age
- Obesity
- History of diabetes mellitus

Patient Outcomes
- Body temperature will be below 100 °F.
- There will be no evidence of infiltrates on CXR.
- Blood, urine, or sputum cultures will be negative.
- Skin, incision(s), and intravenous (IV) and arterial line sites will be free of drainage, erythema, warmth, or tenderness.

Table 13.3 • Teaching Outline: Preoperative Cardiac Surgery

Preparation for Surgery
　Sending important personal belongings home with family or to another
　　secure location
　Shaving (male) or clipping of chest and legs to decrease contamination
　　from skin hair
　Showering
　Surgical consent form
　Administering antianxiety or sleeping medication
　Visit from anesthesiologist at night or in the morning before operation
　Nothing by mouth (NPO) status
　Timing of preoperative sedation
　Availability of chaplains/pastoral care
　Location of intensive care unit, family waiting area, visiting hours

Immediate Postoperative Care and Routines

Cardiac monitor	Central venous pressure line/
Arterial line	hemodynamic monitoring
Epicardial pacing wires	Endotracheal tube and ventilation
Foley catheter	Chest tubes/autotransfusion/
Temperature monitoring	drainage
Arm and thoracic exercises	Nasogastric tube/drainage
Coughing and deep breathing	Analgesia and comfort routines
techniques	

Recovery Phase Care and Routines

Telemetry monitoring	Respiratory care/oxygen delivery
Exercise/activity progression	Weight gain/diuretics
Sleep/rest patterns	Pain/comfort routines
Diet progression	Possible mental or emotional
	changes associated with
	surgery

Nursing Interventions	Rationales
Monitor temperature, CXR, WBC count, and culture results and collaborate with physician on abnormal results.	Elevated temperature and WBC count are expected in the first 72 hr after cardiac surgery, but elevations later suggest infection.
Observe incision(s), skin, IV sites, and mucous membranes for signs/symptoms of infection.	Nonhealing skin, sites, or incision(s) may require further intervention.
Remove invasive lines as soon as indicated.	Lines which bypass the body's first line of defense, the skin, predispose to infection.

Nursing Interventions	**Rationales**
Follow infection control guidelines for care and changing of central lines, peripheral IVs, and epicardial heart wire sites.	
Provide routine incision care daily with soap and water.	Incision care decreases the number of skin bacteria.
Leave incisions open to air after the first 24 hr.	Drainage onto an absorbent pad promotes a moist environment for bacterial growth.
Ambulate patient frequently and encourage position changes.	Activity increases inspiratory effort and mobilizes pulmonary secretions, preventing atelectasis and pneumonia.
Administer respiratory care, incentive spirometry, and coughing and deep breathing exercises every 2 hr while awake.	These activities promote maximal lung capacity and mobilization of respiratory secretions.
Teach patient and family member routine incisional care, daily inspection of incisions, and to notify physician for appearance of redness, swelling, increased tenderness, drainage, warmth at incision or invasive device sites, fever over 101 °F, or yellow/green sputum production.	Wound and pulmonary infections are the most common types of postoperative infections.
Teach patient/family member temperature taking.	

NURSING DIAGNOSIS: HIGH RISK FOR IMPAIRED GAS EXCHANGE

Risk Factors
- Thoracic surgery
- Anesthesia
- Immobility
- Advanced age
- Pain/discomfort
- Preexisting pulmonary disease
- Narcotic analgesics

Patient Outcomes

- Respiratory rate and depth will be within normal limits.
- The CXR will be free of infiltrates, atelectasis, pleural effusion, or pneumothorax.
- Pulse oximetry will exceed 92%.
- Normal activities will be performed without evidence of decompensation.

Nursing Interventions	Rationales
Assess respiratory rate, rhythm, breath sounds, tidal volume, skin color, peripheral temperature, and level of consciousness.	Rate, effort, and volume can be affected by anxiety, pain, and oxygen saturation.
Assess fluid balance: urine output, CXR, edema, weight trend, and breath sounds.	Decreased urine output, prominent pulmonary vessels, presence of edema, weight gain, intake greater than output, and crackles indicate fluid overload which can lead to hypoxia.
Administer diuretics as ordered. Note: If less than desirable response is observed, higher doses or combination of diuretics may be required.	Diuretics decrease pulmonary vascular congestion, improving oxygenation.
Ambulate patient at frequent intervals and encourage patient to change position frequently.	Activity increases physical strength and promotes maximal lung expansion and mobilization of respiratory secretions.
Provide/maintain oxygen delivery system according to parameters.	Supplemental oxygen can enhance circulatory uptake in the lungs.
Add moisture or humidity to oxygen delivery system as needed.	The amount of moisture required will increase during fever or a dry air environment. Moisture can promote free air movement of cilia and maintain protective action of the mucociliary blanket.
Assess/monitor for signs/symptoms of pneumothorax: shortness of breath (SOB), absence of breath sounds at the affected area, cyanosis, crepitus, tracheal deviation, and presence of pneumothorax on CXR.	Pneumothorax may occur as a result of undetected tear in the pleura which allows accumulation of air or gas in the pleural space, collapses the lung, and decreases surface area for diffusion.

Nursing Interventions	Rationales
Assess/monitor for signs/symptoms of atelectasis: crepitant breath sounds, fever, and appearance of atelectasis on CXR.	Atelectasis may occur as a result of incomplete reexplanation of a lung secondary to anesthesia, fluid or secretions.
Assess/monitor for signs/symptoms of pleural effusion: fluid level on percussion, dyspnea, decreased breath sounds on the affected side, cough, increased respiratory effort, and presence of effusion on CXR.	The pleural cavity is often entered during cardiac surgery. Pleural fluid accumulates when it is produced at a rate faster than it is absorbed or drained. Bloody fluid in the pleural cavity is classified as a hemothorax.
Assess/monitor for signs/symptoms of pulmonary embolism: SOB; acute onset of pain which is continuous, "sharp," "stabbing," "like a knife"; pain worse on inspiration, hypoxia; pleural friction rub; tachycardia; tachypnea; and ventilation greater than perfusion on nuclear scan.	Emboli from the deep veins in the legs or pelvis may travel and lodge in a pulmonary arterial vessel via the right side of the heart.
Provide narcotic analgesics to optimize pulmonary work.	Incisional pain interferes with effective coughing and deep breathing.
Monitor respiratory rate and if less than 12/min, consider alternative analgesics and comfort measures.	Morphine can lead to respiratory depression. Narcotic analgesics also suppress the cough reflex, increasing the importance of activity, exercises, and coughing and deep breathing.
Teach patient to continue to do coughing and deep breathing and perform arm and thoracic exercises for 6 weeks. Provide volumetric exerciser for home use. For those with a history of volume overload/congestive heart failure (CHF), instruct in doing a daily weight and recording. Instruct to notify physician of weight gain of 3–5 lbs over 3–5 days. Instruct in the safe use of diuretics/electrolyte supplementation if ordered.	

NURSING DIAGNOSIS: HIGH RISK FOR DECREASED CARDIAC OUTPUT OR HEMODYNAMIC COMPROMISE

Risk Factors
- Dysrhythmias
- Recent cardiac surgery
- Elevated catecholamines
- Electrolyte imbalance
- Fluid overload
- Myocardial ischemia

Patient Outcomes
Patient will have adequate cardiac output, as evidenced by
- normal heart rate and rhythm
- stable blood pressure
- warm, dry skin
- urine output >30 mL/hr

Nursing Interventions	Rationales
Assess/monitor heart rate and rhythm, blood pressure trend, skin temperature, color, presence and quality of peripheral pulses, urine output, and mental status.	Change in heart rate and rhythm can lead to hemodynamic compromise.
Institute pharmacological therapies to increase heart rate when brady-cardia/bradyarrhythmias occur.	Refer to Table 13.4.
Monitor response to therapy and for side effects from therapies.	
Consider other measures to increase heart rate, that is, epicardial ventricular or atrial/ventricular pacing (external).	These leads are sewn to the myocardium at the time of cardiac surgery.
Determine type and location (which cardiac chamber) of epicardial pacing leads.	Right atrial wires are brought out via the skin at the right subcostal area. Right ventricular wires are brought out via the skin at the left subcostal area.
Attach or turn on external pacemaker and generator. Check minimal threshold and adjust pacemaker rate as indicated.	

Nursing Interventions	Rationales
Maintain patient safety while attached to external pacemaker: 1. Occlusive dressing over wires should be dry and intact. 2. When handling pacing wires gloves should be worn. 3. All connections should be secure. 4. Electrical devices in room should be checked for safety.	Stray electricity could travel up the pacing wire and alter cardiac rhythm.
Consider what medications could contribute to a decrease in heart rate and collaborate with physician.	Beta blockers, cardiac glycosides, and calcium channel blockers can cause bradycardia.
Monitor drug levels as indicated.	High levels of antidysrhythmic drugs can cause bradycardia.
Consider other conditions which contribute to a decreased rate and collaborate with physician.	Surgery, ischemia, the Valsalva maneuver, hypovolemia, and hypoxia can cause bradycardia.
Prepare for use of external noninvasive pacemaker, insertion of transveous, transthoracic, or permanent pacemaker as needed.	Permanent damage to the conduction system can result from cardiac surgery, requiring a permanent pacemaker.
Institute pharmacological therapies to decrease heart rate when tachydysrhythmias occur and monitor response.	Refer to Table 13.4.
Consider other factors which contribute to tachydysrhythmias, that is, fever or pain, and institute nursing intervention to achieve normalization of body temperature and physical comfort.	
Confer with physician, administer pharmacological therapies for dysrhythmias, and monitor for side effects.	
Instruct in the safe use of cardiac medications.	Knowing optimal medication schedule and common side effects assists in self-monitoring.
Instruct in pulse counting.	Most antidysrhythmic medications can lead to bradycardia.

Table 13.4 • Dysrhythmias Following Cardiac Surgery

Dysrhythmia	Interventions/Considerations	Medications
Sinus tachycardia	Treat etiology, i.e., fever, pain hypoxia, hypovolemia.	Beta blocker, calcium channel blocker
Sinus bradycardia	Utilize temporary cardiac pacing if hemodynamic compromise	Atropine, isoproterenol (hold medications that can cause bradycardia)
Premature atrial contractions	Assess and intervene if patient is symptomatic.	Digitalis, beta blocker, calcium channel blocker
Atrial tachycardia	Patient is predisposed to ischemia secondary to rapid rate. If hemodynamically unstable and refractory to medications, direct current cardioversion may be required.	Digitalis, procainamide, propanolol, verapamil
Atrial flutter	Vagal stimulation (by physician), rapid atrial pacing, cardioversion.	Digitalis, procainamide, propanolol, verapamil
Atrial fibrillation	Patient may need to be treated to prevent embolization if valve disease or repair/replacement involved. Cardioversion, if unable to convert with medication.	Medications to slow ventricular response and promote conversion to regular rhythm: digitalis, beta blockers, calcium channel blockers, quinidine
Junctional rhythm	Treat etiology, assess if patient is symptomatic, keep external pacemaker on standby.	

Accelerated junctional rhythm	Attempt resumption of sinus or paced rhythm if symptomatic.	
Premature ventricular contractions	Assess electrolyte balance; treat hypokalemia and hypomagnesemia. Ensure adequate oxygenation.	Lidocaine if frequent, paired, triplets, and/or multifocal
Ventricular tachycardia	If symptomatic, precordial thump and electrical cardioversion. If patient is without a pulse, defibrillate immediately.	May require lidocaine, procainamide, and bretyllium for stabilization. Longer term medications include quinidine, procainamide, mexiletine, amiodarone.
Ventricular fibrillation	Defibrillate immediately. Monitor for electrolyte disturbances/hypoxia. Institute hemodynamic support/cardiopulmonary resuscitation when indicated.	Stabilization with pharmacological therapies listed above.
Mobitz I heart block	Assess if patient is symptomatic, increase ventricular rate if symptomatic or hemodynamic compromise; utilize epicardial pacing if indicated.	Atropine; hold digitalis
Mobitz II heart block	Assess if symptomatic with slow ventricular rate; if so, increase ventricular rate as above.	Atropine, isoproterenol
Third-degree heart block	Hemodynamic support/pacing	Isoproterenol

▶

NURSING DIAGNOSIS: ACUTE PAIN

Related To surgical procedure

Defining Characteristics
Moaning
Grimacing
Splinting
Refusal to move

Patient Outcomes
Patient will
- verbalize pain relief and only mild discomfort.
- demonstrate pain is tolerable by ability to have bed and chair mobility.

Nursing Interventions	Rationales
Assess for presence of pain, including location, duration, and severity. Utilize established pain assessment tools and rating scales for accurate assessment.	Knowing the amount and type of pain is necessary to individualize intervention.
Offer and administer analgesics.	
If patient is utilizing morphine sulfate, monitor respiratory rate as a sign of central nervous system (CNS) depression.	Morphine can cause respiratory depression. Narcotic analgesics also supress the cough reflex and slow gastrointestinal motility.
Administer analgesics prior to expected painful experience, that is, arm and shoulder exercises, coughing and deep breathing exercises, and ambulation.	
Provide comfort measures: 1. position changes 2. splinting of incisional area 3. back rubs 4. physical presence 5. restful environment 6. relaxation and distraction techniques	These measures, alone or in combination, can relieve some of the discomfort by reducing painful stimuli and anxiety.

NURSING DIAGNOSIS: KNOWLEDGE DEFICIT

Related To complex treatment regimen

Defining Characteristics

Patient verbalizes inability to manage home care.
There is lack of information on follow-up care.

Patient Outcomes

Patient and/or family members can demonstrate/verbalize elements of self-care in the following areas: incisional care, risk factor modification, physical restrictions, follow-up physician appointments, stress management, outpatient cardiac rehabilitation, diet restriction, medications, physical complications, and emotional changes.

Nursing Interventions	Rationales
Assess misconceptions/misunderstandings of health state.	Misinterpretation or misunderstandings need to be assessed to facilitate accurate clarification of information.
Teach incision care, signs/symptoms of infection, and self-application of antiembolism stockings.	A major focus of the recovery phase is preparation for home.
Teach patient/family member pulse counting and any special parameters related to cardiac medications and activity intolerance.	Discharge planning should include the family as patients may be too ill or fatigued to comprehend all important points.
Teach patient/family member regarding suggested activities at home, per inpatient cardiac rehabilitation recommendations.	Activity recommendations vary according to individual tolerance and other health problems.
Arrange one-to-one or group teaching regarding changes in diet.	
Discuss potential physical complications and postoperative emotional changes with patient and family.	Listing common physical and emotional complications assists with early recognition and early intervention.

Nursing Interventions	Rationales
Provide written information regarding postoperative care and medications, including actions, times of administration, side effects, and special considerations.	Written information will reforce learning by providing a resource to clarify information.
Assist with appointments for follow-up care.	Patients may be unable to make necessary appointments without assistance.

NURSING DIAGNOSIS: HIGH RISK FOR INJURY

Risk Factors
- Abnormal anatomy
- Prosthetic valve

Patient Outcomes
- Patient/family member will demonstrate or verbalize elements of self-care related to prevention of infective endocarditis.
- Patient will remain free of fever, chills, and flulike symptoms associated with endocarditis.

Nursing Interventions	Rationales
Provide patient with written information regarding prevention of endocarditis.	Fatigue or anxiety may interfere with understanding postoperative teaching.
Teach patient/family member regarding normal cardiac anatomy, preoperative defects and surgical correction.	Patient and family need to understand benefits of surgical procedure.
Teach patient/family regarding factors predisposing to endocarditis.	Invasive procedures (surgical, dental) allow entry of bacteria into the blood and can result in endocarditis. See Infective Endocarditis.
Teach patient/family member regarding use of prophylactic antimicrobial agents, what situations require them, and how to obtain them.	It is necessary for patients to alert dental and medical practitioners to their need for prophylactic antibiotics prior to invasive procedures.

Nursing Interventions	Rationales
Teach patient/family member regarding good oral hygiene and other preventive measures against ports of entry.	
Teach patient/family regarding temperature monitoring, parameters of when to contact physician, and signs/symptoms of infective endocarditis.	Early recognition and reporting of fevers, chills, and flulike symptoms lead to early intervention.
Teach patient/family member regarding need for long-term medical identification and to inform all future health care providers with correct information about prosthetic valves and prevention of endocarditis.	

NURSING DIAGNOSIS: HIGH RISK FOR EMBOLIZATION AND BLEEDING

Risk Factors
- Prosthetic heart valve
- Anticoagulant therapy

Patient Outcomes
Patient will
- verbalize need for anticoagulant therapy and indications for use.
- demonstrate understanding of correct and varying dose administration.
- verbalize need for blood tests and medical supervision.
- remain free of thromboembolic or hemorrhagic complications.

Nursing Interventions	Rationales
Explain need for anticoagulant therapy.	Warfarin is prescribed for long-term anticoagulation to prevent thrombi from forming on the prosthetic valve and for chronic atrial fibrillation.
Provide patient/family with medical alert information and identification cards.	Future health care providers will need to be aware of anticoagulation.

Nursing Interventions	Rationales
Instruct in basic action of warfarin (dosage, major side effects), date and time of next PT test, designated physician, and importance of compliance with medication program.	Patients should be informed of the consequences of omission of medication or inadequate follow-up care.
Instruct patient on precautionary measures: 1. no aspirin-containing medications unless specifically prescribed 2. awareness that birth control pills, hormones, and vitamins affect warfarin 3. awareness that alcohol and diet affect warfarin 4. need to carry medical identification 5. measures to prevent physical injury 6. appropriate action should bleeding occur 7. need to inform all physicians and dentists regarding anticoagulation	Precautionary measures prevent complications from anticoagulant therapy.

DISCHARGE PLANNING/CONTINUITY OF CARE:

- Assist with arrangement of follow-up testing and physician appointments.
- Arrange for home care with visiting nurse when indicated.
- Enroll patient in cardiac rehabilitation program.
- Provide with emergency phone numbers.

REFERENCES

Dossey, B. M., & Guzzetta, C. (1992). *Cardiovascular nursing: Holistic practice* (1st ed). St. Louis, MO: Mosby Year Book.

Eagan, J. S., Stewart, S. L., Vitello-Cicciu, J. M. (1991). *Quick reference to cardiac critical care nursing* (1st ed). Rockville, MD: Aspen.

Funk, M., & Pierson, M. G. (1989). Technology versus clinical evaluation for fluid management decisions in CABG patients. *Image: Journal of Nursing Scholarship, winter*, 192–195.

Kern, L. S. (1991). The elderly heart surgery patient. *Critical Care Nursing Clinics of North America, December*, 749–756.

Porth, C. (1990). *Pathophysiology—concepts of altered health states* (3rd ed.). Philadelphia: Lippincott.

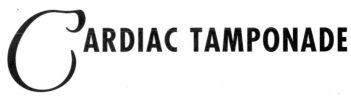

CARDIAC TAMPONADE

Patricia A. Burke, RN, MS, CCRN

Cardiac tamponade occurs when the volume of blood or fluid trapped within the pericardial sac causes intrapericardial pressure to exceed right atrial pressure, compromising diastolic filling. In an intact pericardium, as little as 50 mL of rapidly accumulated pericardial fluid may induce tamponade. In the postoperative cardiovascular surgical patient, mediastinal drainage places the patient at risk, although a larger volume of about 250 mL is required to precipitate tamponade. Slow-growing pericardial effusions allow the pericardium to accommodate as much as 1000 cc of fluid before tamponade occurs. No matter what the volume and circumstances, cardiac tamponade can become an emergency that requires rapid nursing and medical measures to preserve life.

ETIOLOGIES

- Pericarditis with accumulation of pericardial fluid (uremia, malignancy, radiation induced, idiopathic)
- Bleeding into pericardial sac after trauma (gunshot wound, stab wound, motor vehicle accident)
- Bleeding into pericardial sac following invasive procedures (cardiac catheterization, cardiac surgery, endomyocardial biopsy, coronary angioplasty)
- Hemopericardium as complication of anticoagulation
- Suture line disruption following cardiac surgery
- Cardiac or great-vessel rupture

CLINICAL MANIFESTATIONS

- Dyspnea
- Feelings of impending doom or panic
- Lassitude or exertional fatigue (in slow-growing effusion)

CLINICAL/DIAGNOSTIC FINDINGS

- Diminished blood pressure
- Narrowed pulse pressure
- Cardiogenic shock
- Diminished heart sounds
- Muffled pericardial friction rub
- Diminished breath sounds, particularly over left scapula (Ewart's sign)
- Tachypnea
- Tachycardia
- Cool, pale skin
- Pulsus paradoxus (> 10 mmHg difference between inspiratory and expiratory systolic blood pressure)
- Hepatomegaly
- Rising central venous pressure (CVP) > 15 mmHg
- Widened, globular cardiac silhouette on chest xray
- Decreased QRS voltage on the electrogram (ECG), or electrical alternans
- Neck vein distention on inspiration (Kussmaul's sign)
- Echocardiogram: pericardial effusion

NURSING DIAGNOSIS: HIGH RISK FOR DECREASED CARDIAC OUTPUT

Risk Factors
- Distention of pericardial sac with associated rise in intrapericardial pressure
- Impaired right atrial and ventricular filling
- Decreased circulating volume

PATIENT OUTCOMES

- Central venous pressure, mean arterial pressure, and pulse pressure will normalize.
- Heart sounds will be clearly audible on auscultation.
- Neck veins will be flat at 30°–45°.
- The patient will exhibit a normal respiratory pattern and rate.
- Skin will be warm and dry, with pink undertones and pink mucous membranes.
- Peripheral pulses will be palpable and of usual quality.
- Cardiac silhouette will be comparable to pretamponade dimensions on chest x-ray.
- The patient's QRS voltage on the ECG will be comparable to the pretamponade ECG.
- Patient will verbalize/exhibit nonverbal cues that he or she is comfortable.
- Urine output will be at least 30 mL/hr.

Nursing Interventions	**Rationales**
Assess patient for signs and symptoms of hemodynamic instability, such as hypotension, narrowing pulse pressure, new tachycardia, pericardial rub, tachypnea, neck vein distention on inspiration, hepatomegaly, pulsus paradoxus, and pale, cool, skin.	Signs and symptoms of low cardiac output may develop insidiously or suddenly as ventricular filling is compromised.
Assess CVP and ECG changes.	The CVP will rise with impairment of right atrial and ventricular filling. The ECG voltage will decrease with tamponade.
Elicit subjective data from the patient with particular attention to complaints of dyspnea and feelings of "something wrong".	Dyspnea and feelings of impending doom often are associated with low cardiac output.
Prepare for rapid infusion of isotonic intravenous fluids or blood.	When circulating volume is increased, venous pressure will rise to a level greater than that of pericardial pressure and enhance cardiac output until more definitive measures can be taken.
Place patient in high Fowler's position if tolerated.	Elevating the head promotes diaphragmatic excursion but may contribute to hypotension.
Administer oxygen.	Oxygen may relieve dyspnea and enhance PaO_2.
Assure that equipment is available for pericardiocentesis (nonsurgical situation): 50-mL syringe, large-bore spinal needle, lidocaine syringe, chest ECG lead, alligator clamp, and skin prep solution.	Lidocaine provides local anesthetic. Spinal needle and 50-mL syringe aspirate fluid. Alligator clamp attaches chest lead to needle, enabling observation of the ECG.
Have chest-opening equipment available in the intensive care unit (ICU) or triage area for surgical or trauma patient.	Mediastinal opening and exploration must be prompt for relief of hemodynamic compromise. While not ideal to open a patient's chest at bedside, it can become necessary if the patient is profoundly hypotensive or too unstable to take to the operating room.

NURSING DIAGNOSIS: HIGH RISK FOR ALTERED TISSUE PERFUSION—PERIPHERAL

Risk Factors
- Low cardiac output
- Postoperative bleeding
- Deteriorating arterial blood gases
- Falling oxygen transport
- Hemodilution from rapid fluid replacement

Patient Outcomes
- Hemoglobin will measure 11.7–15.7 g/dL (females) or 13.3–17.7 g/dL (males).
- Arterial oxygen saturation will be 90% or greater.
- Capillary refill will be less than 3 s.

Nursing Interventions	Rationales
Monitor hemoglobin and hematocrit and transfuse blood and blood components as prescribed.	Low hemoglobin lessens oxygen transport to tissues and organs.
Assess capillary refill, skin color, temperature, and distal pulses.	Capillary refill greater than 3 s, pale or cyanotic skin, cool skin temperature, and absence of peripheral pulses are indices of poor peripheral perfusion. Rapid infusion of crystalloids predisposes the patient to fluid shifts from rapid decrease in intravascular colloid osmotic pressure and may necessitate diuretic therapy and/or colloid administration.
Assess CVP and pulmonary capillary wedge pressure.	These measurements guide rate of volume replacement.

NURSING DIAGNOSIS: HIGH RISK FOR PATIENT/FAMILY ANXIETY

Risk Factors
- Chest wall pain from accidental or surgical trauma
- Critical illness
- Precipitous nature of tamponade

PATIENT/FAMILY OUTCOMES

- Patient/family will verbalize simple explanations of current problems and treatment.
- Patient will verbalize or nonverbally demonstrate that pain is under control.

Nursing Interventions	Rationales
Offer analgesics at prescribed time intervals and evaluate pain relief and vital signs.	Narcotic analgesics decrease pain and anxiety but may also exacerbate hypotension.
Offer simple explanations of treatment measures to patient and family.	Anticipatory guidance, where possible, eases patient and family anxiety. The degree of anxiety the patient and family are likely to experience makes complex explanations of treatment ineffective; keep explanations simple.

DISCHARGE PLANNING/CONTINUITY OF CARE

- Ensure that patient has basic understanding of the factors contributing to cardiac tamponade.
- If the tamponade was caused by a chronic process, teach the patient signs and symptoms of recurrent pericardial effusion.
- Assist patient to arrange appropriate medical/surgical follow-up.
- Provide instructions regarding prescribed medications, dietary recommendations, and activity.

REFERENCES

Alspach, J. G. (Ed). (1991). *Core curriculum for critical care nursing*. Philadelphia: Saunders.

Guzzetta, C. E., & Dossey, B. M. (1992). *Cardiovascular nursing: Holistic practice*. St. Louis, MO: Mosby Year Book.

Von Rueden, K. T., & Walleck, C. A. (1989). *Advanced critical care nursing*. Rockville, MD: Aspen.

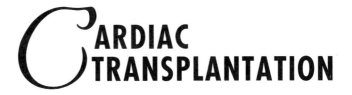

CARDIAC TRANSPLANTATION

Diane K. Dressler, RN, MSN, CCRN, CCTC

Cardiac transplantation is a surgical option for selected patients with end-stage cardiac failure. Orthotopic cardiac transplantation involves replacement of the native heart and is a technology limited by the availability of donor organs. Candidates may be newborn to 65 years old, have recurrent congestive heart failure (CHF), and are thought to have less than 1 year to live. An extensive evaluation is carried out prior to placing patients on a waiting list. Following transplant, 1-year survival is over 80% and 5-year survival over 70%. Patients require careful nursing and medical management during all phases of transplant, from evaluation through long-term follow-up care.

ETIOLOGIES

- Congestive cardiomyopathy: viral, familial, postpartum, idiopathic
- Ischemic cardiomyopathy due to end-stage coronary artery disease
- Failure of other medical and surgical options

CLINICAL MANIFESTATIONS

Preoperative
- Abdominal pain
- Anorexia
- Cachexia
- Cough
- Distended neck veins
- Dyspnea
- Fatigue
- Hepatomegaly
- Hypotension
- Orthopnea
- Pallor and cyanosis

- Palpitations
- Paroxysmal nocturnal dyspnea
- Rales or wheezing
- S_3 gallop
- Syncope
- Weakness

Postoperative
- Patients no longer manifest signs of heart failure unless they are experiencing acute rejection or dysfunction of the transplanted heart.
- Patients do manifest side effects of immunosuppressive drug therapy, which typically consists of cyclosporine, steroids, and azathioprine:
  - arterial hypertension
  - cushingoid changes
  - elevated blood urea nitrogen (BUN) and serum creatinine
  - leukopenia
  - osteoporosis
  - weight gain

CLINICAL/DIAGNOSTIC FINDINGS

Preoperative
- Cardiac catheterization: Diagnostic of cardiac problems not amenable to corrective surgery. Severe fixed pulmonary hypertension (> 4–6 Wood units) may rule out option of transplant.
- Chest x-ray: The heart is massively enlarged and there is pulmonary vascular congestion.
- Electrocardiogram (ECG): Dysrhythmias are common, especially ventricular.
- Echocardiogram: There is severe global hypokinesis of the left ventricle, enlarged cardiac chambers, valvular incompetence, and mural thrombi.
- Endomyocardial biopsy: May define the disease process, such as myocarditis or amyloidosis.
- Liver function tests: These are elevated due to passive liver congestion.
- Nuclear gaited cardiac scan: There are wall motion abnormalities and severe hypokinesis of ventricles with left ventricular ejection fraction 5–20%.
- Psychological testing: Candidates must be free of problems related to compliance, competence, and substance abuse.
- Pulmonary function tests: Often abnormal due to CHF.
- Renal function tests: Often abnormal due to low cardiac output.

Postoperative
- Blood pressure: Moderate to severe hypertension is common.
- Body weight: Obesity and cushingoid features are common.
- Cardiac catheterization: Should show normal coronary arteries. Stenosis may indicate chronic rejection.

- Comblete blood count (CBC): Leukopenia, anemia, and thrombocytopenia may occur from immunosuppressive drugs.
- Chest x-ray: Often shows mild enlargement of transplanted heart.
- Cyclosporine level: Shows serum or blood levels within therapeutic range.
- ECG: Denervated heart may have elevated resting rate. Extra P waves from native atria are not conducted. Delays in conduction such as bundle branch blocks are common.
- Echocardiogram: Should show normal left ventricular ejection fraction without wall motion abnormalities. Mild valvular insufficiency is common.
- Endomyocardial biopsy: Specimens are graded from no acute rejection to severe acute rejection changes.
- Liver function tests: May be mildly elevated due to immunosuppressive drugs.
- Nuclear gaited heart scan: Should show normal ventricular function.
- Renal function tests: BUN and serum creatinine are usually elevated due to cyclosporine nephrotoxicity.

NURSING DIAGNOSIS: HIGH RISK FOR DECREASED CARDIAC OUTPUT

Risk Factors
- Acute rejection
- Chronic rejection
- Decreased myocardial contractility

Patient Outcomes
- Normal cardiac output will be maintained, as evidenced by normal hemodynamic parameters and stable heart rhythm.
- There will be no rejection or resolving rejection on endomyocardial biopsy.

Nursing Interventions	Rationales
Monitor vital signs for hypotension and tachycardia or other dysrhythmias. Note: Resting tachycardia may be normal in the denervated heart.	Patients receiving cyclosporine usually do not have signs of rejection until CHF develops. There may be subtle changes in vital signs or heart rhythm.
Observe for fatigue, dyspnea, edema, and abdominal distress.	Patients should be questioned and examined for signs of CHF.

Nursing Interventions	Rationales
Facilitate scheduling of endomyocardial biopsy when condition has changed.	It is necessary to rule out rejection before working up other potential diagnoses.
Administer augmented immunosuppressive drug therapy as prescribed.	Acute rejection is often treated with large doses of steroids.
Observe for increasing hemodynamic instability: blood pressure (BP) < 90 mmHg, right atrial pressure (RAP) > 15 mmHg, pulmonary capillary wedge pressure (PCWP) > 15 mmHg, oliguria, rales, and dyspnea.	Acute rejection can progress to cardiogenic shock. Patient may require transfer to critical care unit.
Administer inotropic agents and manage ventilatory support and mechanical circulatory assistance as necessary.	Most patients respond to therapy and may recover normal heart function.
Instruct patient to report signs and symptoms of cardiac problems.	Early reporting of cardiac problems facilitates prompt treatment, avoiding crises.

NURSING DIAGNOSIS: HIGH RISK FOR INJURY

Risk Factors
- Serial endomyocardial biopsies

Patient Outcomes
- Following endomyocardial biopsy procedures, the patient will demonstrate stable hemodynamics, as evidenced by systolic blood pressure above 100 and heart rate 60–110.
- The ECG will show normal sinus rhythm.
- There will be no evidence of bleeding.
- There will be no evidence of hemothorax or pneumothorax.

Nursing Interventions	Rationales
Hold anticoagulant therapy prior to procedure.	Although the biopsy catheter is passed through a vein, bleeding complications are possible.

Nursing Interventions	Rationales
Observe jugular or femoral site for bleeding, apply pressure prn.	Application of pressure will minimize bleeding and prevent hematoma formation.
Assess blood pressure, heart rate, and peripheral perfusion every 15 min for 1 hr, then every hour for 4 hr.	Hypotension and dysrhythmia may result from bioptome trauma to the endocardium. Perforation and tamponade are rare complications.
Assess respiratory rate, depth, pattern, and symmetry of breath sounds every 15 min for 1 hr, then every hour for 4 hr.	Hemothorax and pneumothorax are rare complications.
Limit activity as prescribed, usually bedrest with head of bed elevated for 2–4 hr postprocedure.	This minimizes bleeding complications.

NURSING DIAGNOSIS: HIGH RISK FOR INFECTION

Risk Factors
- Immunosuppressed state
- Exposure to hospital environment
- Invasive diagnostic procedures or treatments

Patient Outcomes
- The patient will be free from infection, as evidenced by
  - normal wound healing
  - body temperature < 99°F
  - no nasal congestion or cough
  - no chills
  - no vomiting or diarrhea
  - no urinary tract symptoms
  - normal white blood cell (WBC) count
  - no infiltrate on chest x-ray
  - negative sputum, urine, and blood cultures
- The skin and mucous membranes will remain intact.
- Exposure to virulent organisms will be limited.

Nursing Interventions	Rationales
Observe incisions, intravenous (IV) sites, pacemaker wire sites, skin, and mucous membranes for signs of infection.	Therapeutic immunosuppression increases the risk of infection.

Nursing Interventions	Rationales
Report temperature above 99°F, cough, infiltrate on chest x-ray, and altered WBC and differential counts and culture reports to physician.	The most common site of serious infection is the lungs, but upper respiratory, urinary tract, oral, gastrointestinal, and skin infections also occur.
Observe for subtle signs of infection such as malaise.	Patients receiving steroids may not show typical signs of infection.
Insert indwelling lines and tubes under sterile conditions, maintain aseptically, and discontinue as soon as possible. Avoid rectal temperatures and enemas.	The skin and mucous membranes are the first line of defense against infection.
Use meticulous hand washing before and after patient contact.	Good hand washing is thought to be the most important strategy to prevent transmissible infection.
Use modified protective isolation with private room and masks for intensively immunosuppressed patients.	Infection is usually derived from endogenous flora and ubiquitous organisms in the environment.
Prohibit contact with persons having upper respiratory tract infection, diarrhea, open wound, and skin infection.	Exposure to infectious organisms must be limited.
Minimize the time the patient is in the intensive care unit (ICU) and in the hospital.	There is increased risk of exposure to pathogenic organisms in the hospital environment.
Instruct patient to report signs and symptoms of infection.	Early diagnosis and treatment of infection are imperative in immunosuppressed patients.

NURSING DIAGNOSIS: HIGH RISK FOR RENAL DYSFUNCTION AND HYPERTENSION

Risk Factors
- Cyclosporine therapy and associated nephrotoxicity

Patient Outcomes
The patient will demonstrate stable renal function and blood pressure, as evidenced by

- BUN < 30 mg/dL
- serum creatinine < 1.5 mg/dL
- stable body weight
- normal urine output
- therapeutic cyclosporine level
- systolic BP < 140 mmHg
- diastolic BP < 90 mmHg

Nursing Interventions	Rationales
Monitor BUN, serum creatinine, daily weight, and urine output and compare to patient's normal values.	The most common side effect of cyclosporine is nephrotoxicity, and the majority of transplant patients have elevated BUN and serum creatinine levels.
Monitor blood pressure and administer antihypertensive agents as prescribed.	Arterial hypertension is seen in most patients on cyclosporine and may further compromise renal function.
Monitor serum or whole blood trough cyclosporine levels.	High drug levels promote renal dysfunction and high blood pressure.
Avoid administration of other nephrotoxic agents such as contrast, nonsteroidal anti-inflammatory drugs, and some antibiotics.	Additive nephrotoxicity occurs with these agents.
Ensure adequate hydration and monitor renal function if nephrotoxic drugs are administered.	Hydration minimizes nephrotoxicity.
Teach patients to report weight gain, decreased urine output, and hypertension.	Early intervention with these problems can minimize long-term complications. Home blood pressure monitoring aids assessment.

NURSING DIAGNOSIS: FLUID VOLUME EXCESS

Related To corticosteroid therapy

Defining Characteristics
Edema
Hyperglycemia
Hypokalemia
Weight gain

Patient Outcomes

Fluid and electrolyte balance will be maintained, as evidenced by
- stable body weight
- balanced intake and output
- serum potassium 3.5–5.0 mEq/L
- fasting blood sugar < 140 mg/100 mL

Nursing Interventions	Rationales
Measure daily weight and intake and output. Assess for edema.	Steroids cause fluid retention, edema, increased appetite, and weight gain, especially at high doses.
Monitor electrolytes and administer potassium supplement as indicated.	Steroids may cause hypokalemia.
Monitor blood sugar and report consistent elevation for evaluation and treatment.	Steroid-induced diabetes occurs in some patients.
Adjust IV fluids; adjust dietary restrictions collaboratively with physician and dietician.	Needs for dietary restriction of sodium and fluids and for potassium replacement change over time.
Instruct patient and family on dietary recommendations.	Most patients are instructed to follow a low-cholesterol, no-added-salt, limited-calorie diet.
Assure patient that fluid retention and weight gain usually decrease over time.	Setroid doses are usually lowered over time.

NURSING DIAGNOSIS: HIGH RISK FOR BONE MARROW SUPPRESSION

Risk Factors
- Azathioprine therapy

Patient Outcomes

The patient will demonstrate stable bone marrow function, as evidenced by
- WBC > 4,000/mm^3
- hemoglobin > 12 g/dL
- hematocrit > 38%
- platelet count > 130,000/mm^3

Nursing Interventions	Rationales
Monitor CBC and compare to patient's normal values.	Bone marrow suppression is a possible side effect of azathioprine.
Report leukopenia or other low values to physician.	White blood cells are usually affected first because of their short survival.
Hold azathioprine for WBC under 4,000/mm³.	Leukopenia increases susceptibility to infection. In patients with persistent low counts, the drug is discontinued.

NURSING DIAGNOSIS: HIGH RISK FOR INEFFECTIVE FAMILY COPING

Risk Factors
- Complex illness
- Postoperative complications
- Multiple stressors and demands occurring simultaneously

Patient/Family Outcomes
- The patient and family will verbalize understanding of complications.
- The patient and family will demonstrate a positive attitude toward future health.
- The family will serve as source of patient support.

Nursing Interventions	Rationales
Assess patient and family for anxiety, depression, hostility, fear, or other indicators of compromised coping.	Problems of rejection, infection, and complications of drugs are common following transplant and may be difficult to cope with.
Explain physiological changes that predispose transplant patients to complications.	Understanding the reasons behind problems decreases feelings of lack of control.
Emphasize that other patients have survived these problems.	Maintaining hope enhances coping.
Suggest strategies the patient can use to assist in recovery and maintaining future health.	Patients have control over some complications but not over others.

Nursing Interventions	Rationales
Establish a primary nurse spokesperson with patient and family representative to promote consistent communication and emotional support.	Consistent and frequent communication related to patient problems and progress enhances coping.
Refer patient or family for professional counseling if indicated.	Therapeutic discussions with physicians and nurses are helpful to most families, but occasionally families need referral to cope with fear of future complications.

NURSING DIAGNOSIS: HIGH RISK FOR BODY IMAGE DISTURBANCE

Risk Factors
- Cushingoid changes
- Emotional instability

Patient Outcomes
The patient will:
- acknowledge changes in body appearance and express feelings of positive self-worth.
- adopt lifestyle changes which minimize physical changes.

Nursing Interventions	Rationales
Discuss posttransplant physical changes with patient to assess feelings about body image.	Cushingoid changes such as weight gain, moon facies, acne, fragile skin, protuberant abdomen, and thin extremities may affect body image.
Discuss posttransplant emotional changes with patient to assess self-concept.	Steroids may cause mood swings and emotional instability. Other patients struggle to integrate donor identity and imagine they assume donor traits.
Employ a team approach to manage problems.	Steroid reduction when possible, dietary counseling, cardiac rehabilitation, and psychological counseling may be helpful.

Nursing Interventions	Rationales
Invite patient to transplant support group meetings.	Support groups provide emotional support and a forum to exchange information on coping with common problems.

NURSING DIAGNOSIS: KNOWLEDGE DEFICIT

Related To complex treatment plan

Defining Characteristics
Verbalization indicating inadequate understanding of or ability to perform desired health behaviors

Patient Outcomes
The patient and family will verbalize and demonstrate knowledge related to
- recognition and prevention of infection
- recognition and prevention of rejection
- complications of immunosuppressive drugs
- lifestyle recommendations
- routine follow-up care

Nursing Interventions	Rationales
Assess patient and family knowledge related to self-care.	Transplant patients need detailed information to manage self-care, and teaching is done over time, continuing during outpatient care.
Review information outlined in a cardiac transplant teaching plan (Table 15.1).	Accurate information enables patients to assume responsibility for themselves and enhances compliance. The ability to recognize and report problems before they become life threatening is essential.
Provide discharge booklet or written instructions.	Information provided verbally during times of stress is often not retained.

Table 15.1 • Heart Transplant Teaching Plan

The patient and family will:

1. Verbalize information related to immunosuppressive drugs:
   a. Common side effects
   b. Timing of doses
   c. Laboratory measurement of cyclosporine levels
   d. Adequate supply of medications

2. Demonstrate accuracy on self-administration of medications:
   a. Cyclosporine
   b. Azathioprine
   c. Prednisone
   d. Other prescribed medications

3. Verbalize strategies to prevent infection:
   a. Avoiding people with infection
   b. Careful dietary choices

4. List signs and symptoms of infection and when to call physician:
   a. Fever > 100°F
   b. Cough, sore throat, nasal congestion
   c. Nausea, vomiting, diarrhea
   d. Cutaneous and oral lesions

5. Verbalize strategies to prevent rejection:
   a. Take medications exactly as directed.
   b. Notify transplant team of changes in medications.
   c. Avoid alcohol and over-the-counter drugs.

6. Verbalize possible signs and symptoms of rejection:
   a. Signs of congestive heart failure
   b. Hypotension
   c. Dysrhythmias

7. Accurately record vital signs and weight daily:
   a. Record keeping
   b. Knowledge of acceptable parameters

8. Verbalize guidelines for low-cholesterol, no-added-salt diet:
   a. Maintaining body weight within recommended parameters
   b. Balancing intake with activity

9. Demonstrate compliance with activity and exercise recommendations:
   a. Progressive cardiac rehabilitation
   b. Returning to work or normal activities

10. Demonstrate knowledge of routine follow-up care:
    a. Laboratory work and clinic visit
    b. Endomyocardial biopsy schedule
    c. Yearly full-heart catheterization

11. Verbalize satisfaction with posttransplant recovery:
    1. Management of emotional problems
    b. Stress management
    c. Transplant support group

▼

DISCHARGE PLANNING/CONTINUITY OF CARE

- Begin discharge planning early as cardiac transplant patients go home as soon as possible because of increased risk of infection in the hospital environment.
- Facilitate communication with the clinical transplant coordinator and physicians who will manage follow-up care.
- Assist with appointments for clinic visits, laboratory tests, and endomyocardial biopsy.
- Consult a social worker to assist with transportation problems which may interfere with follow-up care.
- Consult a financial counselor to assist with insurance problems related to hospitalization or prescription medication.

REFERENCES

Baumgartner, W. A., Reitz, B. A., & Achuff, S. C. (1990). *Heart and heart-lung transplantation.* Philadelphia: Saunders.

Guzzetta, C. E., & Dossey, B. M. (1992). *Cardiovascular nursing: Holistic practice.* St. Louis, MO: Mosby Year Book.

Muirhead, J. (1992). Heart and heart-lung transplantation. *Critical Care Nursing Clinics of North America, 4*(1), 97–109.

O'Connell, J. B., Bourge, R. C., Constanzo-Nordin, M. R., Driscoll, D. J., Morgan, J. P., Rose, E. A., & Utretsky, B. F. (1992). Cardiac transplantation: Recipient selection, donor procurement, and medical follow-up. *Circulation, 86*(3), 1061–1079.

Smith, S. L. (1990). *Tissue and organ transplantation.* St. Louis, MO: Mosby Year Book.

▼

$\mathcal{A}$ORTIC ANEURYSM REPAIR

Julie A. Sommer, RN, MSN

An aneurysm is a weakening and ballooning out of an arterial wall. The term *aneurysm* is used to describe all enlarged areas of the arterial system that have the potential to rupture. Aneurysms may be fusiform (a spindle-shaped enlargement involving the entire aortic circumference), saccular (an outpouching of the arterial wall with a narrowed neck), or dissecting (a hemorrhagic separation in the aortic wall, where blood flows down between layers of the arterial wall). Thoracic aneurysms are an abnormal widening of the ascending, transverse, or descending portion of the thoracic aorta. Abdominal aortic aneurysms occur in the abdominal aorta between the renal arteries and iliac branches and are seen most commonly. Treatment for this condition may involve medical therapy (controlling hypertension) for small aneurysms or those too extensive to repair or surgical therapy. Aneurysms are repaired using a Dacron graft to replace the diseased section of the aorta. The involved vessels along the aortic wall may need to be reimplanted into the graft. For example, repair of an ascending aortic aneurysm involves reimplantation of the coronary arteries. Abdominal aortic aneurysm surgery utilizes a tube graft or Y-shaped graft that is stitched to the aorta proximally and the lower aorta or iliac arteries distally.

ETIOLOGIES

- Atherosclerosis
- Cystic medial necrosis: a hereditary condition that affects the middle lining of the arterial walls and predisposes to development of aneurysms along the aorta
- Marfan's syndrome: a hereditary condition that affects connective tissue and predisposes to development of aneurysms along the aorta
- Aging
- Hypertension
- Blunt trauma
- Smoking
- Obesity

CLINICAL MANIFESTATIONS

- Ascending aneurysms that involve the aortic valve
  - aortic insufficiency
  - diastolic murmur
  - chest pain similar to angina
  - congestive heart failure
- Arch aneurysms
  - chest pain
  - pulsation above the suprasternal notch
  - difference in blood pressure between the right and left upper extremities
  - neurological changes: confusion, decreased level of consciousness
  - tracheal deviation
  - dyspnea
  - coughing
  - hemoptysis
  - wheezing
  - hoarseness
- Abdominal aneurysms
  - back pain
  - abdominal pain
  - pulsation along the abdominal aorta
- Aortic dissections
  - chest pain: sudden sharp knifelike, ripping, tearing pain that does not radiate

CLINICAL/DIAGNOSTIC FINDINGS

- Pulsatile mass on physical examination
- Chest x-ray may show tracheal deviation, widened mediastinum, or a large mediastinal mass in thoracic aneurysms.
- Ultrasound of the abdomen will define dimensions of abdominal aneurysm and whether it contains clot.
- Computerized tomography (CT) scan of the chest shows dimensions of thoracic aneurysm.
- Computerized tomography scan of the abdomen shows dimensions of abdominal aneurysm.
- Cardiac catheterization with aortogram determines the origin and extent of the aneurysm, the size of a false lumen if present, and whether the aortic valve is affected.

NURSING DIAGNOSIS: HIGH RISK FOR ALTERED TISSUE PERFUSION—SYSTEMIC

Risk Factors
- Major vascular surgery
- Hypertension
- Hypothermia

Patient Outcomes
The patient will have adequate systemic perfusion as evidenced by
- blood pressure maintained at 100–140 mmHg systolic and 60–90 mmHg diastolic
- temperature at 98°F within 6 hr of surgery
- urine output > 30 mL/hr
- adequate neurovascular sensation and movement
- peripheral pulses present and strong
- orientation to time, place, and person

Nursing Interventions	Rationales
Monitor vital signs for hypertension, hypotension, and labile blood pressure.	Aortic cross-clamping and vascular trauma increases peripheral vascular resistance and may increase blood pressure. Intraoperative and postoperative volume loss can lead to hypotension.
Titrate intravenous vasodilator agents, such as sodium nitroprusside, as prescribed to maintain normotension (usual dosage: sodium nitroprusside 0.5–8.0 μg/kg/min.)	Hypertension stretches vascular suture lines and can result in increased bleeding.
Assess skin temperature, color, and capillary refill hourly.	Poor peripheral perfusion is an early indicator of hypovolemia or circulatory shock. Cyanotic areas on toes may indicate microemboli.
Assess peripheral pulses for strength and compare to preoperative parameters.	Absence of peripheral pulses may indicate complications from abdominal aortic aneurysm surgery such as major emboli.

Nursing Interventions	**Rationales**
Assess color and quantity of urine output every hour.	Patients undergoing abdominal aortic aneurysm resection are at risk of renal failure secondary to preoperative renal insufficiency, inadequate hydration, hypotension, or atheromatous embolization to the renal arteries.
Assess neurological status hourly: level of consciousness, strength, and movement of extremities.	Paraplegia may occur due to inadequate spinal cord perfusion from aortic cross-clamping, hypotension, or both during the surgery. There is also a risk of embolic cerebrovascular accident (CVA) during vascular surgery.
Monitor electrocardiogram (ECG) and assess for signs of ischemia, ST elevation, T-wave inversion, or premature ventricular contractions (PVCs).	The high incidence of coronary disease in patients with aortic aneurysms, preexisting hypertension, stress of surgery, and altered tissue perfusion contribute to the potential for coronary ischemia and myocardial infarction.
Monitor core body temperature and rewarm slowly with warming mattress and blankets.	Hypothermia causes increased vasoconstriction resulting in hypertension.

NURSING DIAGNOSIS: HIGH RISK FOR FLUID VOLUME DEFICIT

Risk Factors
- Major vascular surgery
- Cardiopulmonary bypass for repair of ascending aorta and aortic arch
- Postoperative bleeding

Patient Outcomes
- Central venous pressure (CVP) 6–8 mmHg and pulmonary capillary wedge pressure (PCWP) 6–12 mmHg will be maintained.
- Equal or positive fluid balance and stable body weight will be maintained.
- Hemoglobin and hematocrit will be within normal limits.
- Patient will maintain an equal or positive fluid balance and stable body weight.

- Thoracic aortic aneurysm surgery:
  - Mediastinal drainage will be below 100 mL/hr.
  - There are no signs or symptoms of cardiac tamponade.
- Abdominal aortic aneurysm surgery:
  - Abdominal girth will not enlarge.

Nursing Interventions	Rationales
Monitor CVP and PCWP continuously according to postoperative orders.	Low circulating blood volume is evidenced by low CVP and PCWP.
Monitor intake (IV, PO, and medications) and output (urine and other drainage).	Decreased urine output may indicate hemorrhage, hypovolemia, or renal insufficiency.
Monitor laboratory data: complete blood count (CBC), prothrombin time (PT), partial thromboplastin time (PTT), and electrolytes.	Falling hemoglobin and hematocrit and abnormal coagulation parameters can indicate hemorrhage.
Weigh daily.	
Administer colloids, crystalloids, or blood products as prescribed.	Large amounts of IV fluid may be required to maintain intravascular volume caused by "third spacing" secondary to major vascular surgery.
Monitor amount of mediastinal drainage (thoracic aneurysm surgery).	Increased mediastinal drainage can indicate hemorrhage.
Assess for signs and symptoms of cardiac tamponade (thoracic aneurysm surgery): 1. equalization of right- and left-sided heart pressures 2. high CVP 3. hypotension	Cardiac tamponade (compression of the heart by fluid within the pericardium) restricts the heart's ability to fill and produces increased systemic and pulmonary venous pressure and decreased cardiac output. Early recognition decreases mortality.
Measure abdominal girth daily (abdominal aortic aneurysm surgery).	An increase in abdominal girth is an early indication of hemorrhage.

NURSING DIAGNOSIS: HIGH RISK FOR INEFFECTIVE AIRWAY CLEARANCE

Risk Factors
- Endotracheal intubation
- Impaired mucociliary clearance related to anesthesia
- Nonventilation during cardiopulmonary bypass

Patient Outcomes
- The endotracheal tube will remain in correct position, as evidenced by auscultation of both lung fields.
- Adequate oxygenation and ventilation will be maintained, as evidenced by respiratory rate 12–24, pulse 60–100, and arterial blood gases (ABGs) and/or pulse oximetry within normal limits.

Nursing Interventions	Rationales
Auscultate breath sounds upon admission and hourly.	Auscultation is necessary to verify placement of endotracheal tube.
Assess and record indicators of oxygenation and ventilatory status: ABGs, pulse oximetry, respiratory rate, and level of consciousness (LOC).	
Assess rhythm, rate, and depth of respirations every hour.	
Monitor color of skin and nail beds.	Pallor and cyanosis are indicators of hypoxemia.
Monitor oxygen saturation by oximetry.	
Adjust and maintain ventilator settings according to unit protocol.	Ventilation and oxygenation needs may change frequently in the immediate postoperative period.
Suction prn while intubated and cough and deep breathe every hour after extubation.	Inhalation anesthesia and hypoventilation during anesthesia can precipitate atelectasis and production of thick secretions.

Nursing Interventions	Rationales
Administer hand-held nebulizer or intermittent positive pressure breathing (IPPB) with or without albuterol as ordered.	Patients who are at high risk for respiratory complications postoperatively require vigorous pulmonary intervention.
Encourage early ambulation and change position in bed frequently.	Ambulation and frequent position changes mobilize secretions.

NURSING DIAGNOSIS: HIGH RISK FOR INFECTION

Risk Factors
- Surgical procedure
- Artificial material in surgical graft
- Invasive monitoring lines

Patient Outcomes
Patient will be free of infection, as evidenced by
- normal wound healing
- body temperature < 99 °F
- absence of chills
- normal white blood cell (WBC) count

Nursing Interventions	Rationales
Assess surgical wound site. Cleanse with soap and water, or antibacterial agent as prescribed.	Cleansing wounds decreases the growth of surface bacteria.
Monitor body temperature.	
Monitor lab values: CBC and differential count.	Leukocytosis and a "shift to the left" indicative of many immature WBCs (bands or stabs) are indicators of infection.
Cover incision site during invasive procedures such as suctioning.	Covering the wound protects the incision site from bacterial invasion from secretions.
Remove invasive lines such as IVs, Foley catheters, and nasogastric (NG) tubes as soon as possible after surgery.	Invasive lines can lead to infection by bypassing the body's natural protection from the skin and mucous membranes.
Use Universal Precautions with all contact involving body fluids.	

NURSING DIAGNOSIS: ACUTE PAIN

Related To surgical incision

Defining Characteristics
Verbalization of pain
Restlessness and agitation
Facial mask of pain
Splinting of pain site
Inability to concentrate

Patient Outcomes
The patient will be pain free, as evidenced by
- verbalization of comfort
- freely coughing and deep breathing

Nursing Interventions	Rationales
Assess pain location and intensity.	The amount of pain can vary considerably between individuals.
Administer pain medication every 1–2 hr.	Patients who have recently undergone surgery will usually experience intense surgical discomfort for the first few days.
Maintain proper body alignment. Teach relaxation and distraction techniques. Splint incisional area during exercises.	
Medicate prior to any activity or painful procedures: removal of chest tubes and ambulation.	Timing of pain medications is most effective if the medication effect peaks during the period of highest pain.
Administer epidural anesthesia as prescribed.	Epidural anesthesia is frequently used for aneurysm surgery. Patients are able to ambulate and cough and deep breathe with minimal discomfort.

NURSING DIAGNOSIS: HIGH RISK FOR ALTERED NUTRITION—LESS THAN BODY REQUIREMENTS

Risk Factors
- NPO status
- Decreased gastrointestinal (GI) motility
- Fatigue
- Pain

Patient Outcomes
- Nutritional intake will be adequate to maintain a positive nitrogen balance.
- Body weight will be stable.
- Surgical wounds will heal normally.

Nursing Interventions	Rationales
Assess nutritional status, including weight, appetite, usual eating patterns, and nutrients needed for wound healing.	A positive nitrogen balance promotes wound healing.
Assess GI function. Auscultate for bowel sounds and initiate PO intake as soon as GI motility resumes (often 4–5 days for abdominal aortic aneurysm patient).	Oral intake is the preferred source of nutritional intake when the GI tract is functioning.
Monitor serum prealbumin at regular intervals.	This provides current information about nutritional status.
Medicate the patient for pain.	When patients are in pain, their appetite decreases.
Provide small, frequent meals.	
Provide for rest periods before meals and maintain a quiet, unhurried environment.	
When oral intake is poor, conduct calorie count for 3 days and collaborate with dietitian to determine nutritional goals.	
Have dietary personnel plan menus that include individual food preferences.	

Nursing Interventions	Rationales
Collaborate with physician regarding enteral or total parental nutrition (TPN) when unable to resume oral intake after 4–5 days.	

NURSING DIAGNOSIS: KNOWLEDGE DEFICIT

Related To surgical recovery

Defining Characteristics

Verbalization indicating inadequate understanding of postoperative regimen.

Patient Outcomes

The patient will verbalize and demonstrate knowledge related to
- postoperative coughing and deep breathing
- pain management
- incision care
- early ambulation

Nursing Interventions	Rationales
Assess knowledge about postoperative recovery preoperatively.	Preoperative assessment of knowledge provides a starting point for teaching.
Explain postoperative recovery, including coughing and deep breathing, pain management, incision care, and early ambulation. Provide written instructions.	Patients retain information better if two teaching methods are used.
Have the patient demonstrate coughing and deep breathing techniques.	It is easier to cough and deep breathe prior to surgery.
Answer any questions.	

DISCHARGE PLANNING/CONTINUITY OF CARE

- Patients are discharged from the hospital in 7–10 days.
- A low-cholesterol, low-salt diet is encouraged.
- Smokers are advised to quit smoking.
- Incision care instructions are provided.
- Body temperature is monitored. A fever above 100 °F and/or shaking chills should be reported.
- Most patients may begin driving in 2–4 weeks following discharge.
- Lifting restriction of more than 10 lb for 6 weeks is recommended.
- Medical follow-up with the surgeon is needed in 2–4 weeks following discharge.
- Social workers or discharge planners assist patients who have special discharge needs or financial concerns.

REFERENCES

Barringer, T. (1991). Ascending aortic arch aneurysms and dissections: Discussion and nursing management. *Progress in Cardiovascular Nursing*, 6(1), 13–20.

Cisar, N., & Pifarre, R. (1990). Traumatic descending thoracic aneurysms: Discussion and nursing care. *Progress in Cardiovascular Nursing*, 5(1), 13–20.

Clochesy, J. M., Breu, C., Cardin, S., Rudy, E. G., & Whittaker, A. A. (1993). *Critical care nursing*. Philadelphia: Saunders.

Gettrust, K. V., & Brabec, P. D. (1992). *Nursing diagnosis in clinical practice*. Albany, NY: Delmar.

▼

Cardiovascular Electronic/Assistive Devices

▼

ARTIFICIAL CARDIAC PACING

Linda M. Lundin, RN

Cardiac pacing is a means of producing an electrical stimulus to the heart when the person's own conduction system has failed. The pacing system, whether it is permanent or temporary, is an electrical circuit that consists of a power source (battery, generator) and a lead (electrode) that transport the energy or electrical impulse to the cardiac cells resulting in depolarization. The stimulus may occur through electrodes endocardially or epicardially. The leads may be placed epicardially at the time of open heart surgery or endocardially by means of a transvenous approach using local anesthesia. The most common site for transvenous insertion is subclavian or jugular.

Another means of temporary pacing is external transthoracic pacing or transcutaneous pacing (TP). This type of pacing is accomplished by placing large surface skin electrodes, 5–10 cm in diameter, in the anterior and posterior positions, connected to external pacing sources that can provide high voltage output up to 200 milliamperes (mA). Usually an output of 55–90 mA is adequate for capture, while internal pacing only requires 5 mA. External pacing is used when transvenous pacing is not readily available or until transvenous pacing can be initiated.

ETIOLOGIES

Etiological factors for conduction disturbances such as asystole, bradycardia, or atrioventricular (AV) block include but are not limited to

- acute anterior or anteroseptal myocardial infarction (MI) resulting in ischemia in the intraventricular septum
- inferior or posterolateral MI resulting in ischemia to the sinoatrial (SA) or AV node
- sinus node dysfunction
- cardiac drug toxicity (e.g., digitalis, potassium, quinidine, procainamide, beta-adrenergic blockers)
- electrolyte imbalance (e.g., hyperkalemia, hypocalcemia)

- infectious diseases (e.g., scarlet fever, measles, tuberculosis, and syphilis)
- induction of anesthesia (can increase preexisting block)
- cardiac surgery (causing edema, inflammation, or damage around conduction system)
- calcified valvular heart disease
- sclerodegenerative disease of conduction system
- congenital heart block
- coronary artery disease causing ischemia to sinus or AV node

CLINICAL MANIFESTATIONS

- Dizziness
- Syncope
- Fatigue
- Weakness
- Altered level of consciousness
- Angina
- Hypotension
- Ventricular dysrhythmias
- Shortness of breath
- Dyspnea
- Decreased urine output
- Heart failure

CLINICAL/DIAGNOSTIC FINDINGS

Twelve-lead ECG and/or Holter monitor
- Bradydysrhythmias
  - Sinus pauses or arrest
  - Sinus bradycardias
  - Slow junctional rhythms
  - Idioventricular rhythms
- Heart block
  - Second-degree AV block (Mobitz II)
  - Third-degree AV block
- Atrial fibrillation or flutter with a slow ventricular response
- Tachydysrhythmias that are unresponsive to drug therapy (purpose of pacing would be to overdrive rhythm)

Electrophysiology testing
- "Sick sinus" syndrome: (prolonged sinus node recovery time)
- Identification of retrograde conduction or accessory pathways causing supraventricular tachycardias
- Identification of prolongation or block of atrioventricular conduction

NURSING DIAGNOSIS: HIGH RISK FOR DECREASED CARDIAC OUTPUT

Risk Factors
- Bradydysrhythmias
- Conduction abnormalities
- Pacemaker malfunction
- Pacemaker syndrome
- Pacemaker-mediated dysrhythmias

Patient Outcomes
Patient will maintain stable hemodynamic status, as evidenced by
- electrocardiogram (ECG) with normal functioning pacemaker
- ECG will be free of ventricular ectopy
- systolic pressure > 90 mmHg
- urine output > 30 mL/hr
- absence of
  - decreased tissue perfusion
  - weakness
  - decreased level of consciousness
  - fatigue
  - syncope
  - angina
  - shortness of breath (SOB)
  - dyspnea
  - ventricular dysrhythmias

Nursing Interventions	Rationales
Monitor vital signs every 15 min postimplant or until stable, then every 30 min for 1 hr, then every 4 hr for 24 hr, then twice daily.	Decreased blood pressure may occur after a pacemaker procedure due to sedation, malfunctions, or pacemaker syndrome. Pacemaker syndrome presents itself as lightheadedness, SOB, syncope, and hypotension. It develops when there is a loss of the activation sequence of the heart in which the atria contract first and then after an appropriate delay, the ventricles contract (AV synchrony). Asynchrony leads to decreased ventricular filling and therefore decreased cardiac output (CO).

Nursing Interventions	Rationales
Monitor ECG rhythm continuously postimplantation for malfunctions (see Table 17.1): 1. noncapture 2. nonsensing 3. nonfiring	Continuous monitoring is needed to detect malfunctions that may lead to bradyarrhythmias and decreased CO.
Monitor ECG rhythm continuously for ventricular dysrhythmias and treat appropriately with prescribed medications such as lidocaine.	Pacer leads, especially immediately postimplantation, may cause frequent ventricular dysrhythmias leading to decreased CO.
Interpret ECG rhythms by knowing mode of pacemaker, measuring rate, and measuring appropriate intervals (see Tables 17.2–17.4).	Proper interpretation will detect pacer malfunction.
Maintain patient on bedrest first 24–48 hr postimplant with activity restrictions for affected extremity, that is, do not raise arm over head if pacemaker insertion is brachial, subclavian, or jugular. Do not bend or raise leg if pacer is in femoral area. Turn to the left side only.	Excessive activity postimplantation may dislodge the lead, causing pacer malfunction or ventricular irritability and dysrhythmias. Turning to the right side may cause the lead to dislodge.
Protect from microshocks in temporary pacemakers by taking the following precautions: 1. Cover exposed lead ends with rubber glove and secure with tape. 2. Wear rubber gloves when handling pacer leads. 3. Have all electrical equipment used on or near the patient checked for proper grounding.	Static electricity from people and stray electrical current from equipment can travel down the lead, causing tachyarrhythmias or myocardial damage.

Nursing Interventions	Rationales
4. Place a sign over the patient's bed that reads "Temporary Pacemaker—Electrical Safety Precautions." 5. Avoid applying two different line-powered electrical devices to the patient at the same time. 6. Do not touch pacer lead while touching electrical devices. 7. Do not change batteries of the generator while the generator is hooked to patient. 8. Disconnect temporary pacer before defibrillation.	
Monitor patient for signs and symptoms of tamponade, including hypotension, increased venous pressures, pulsus paradoxus, and muffled heart tones.	Perforation of the ventricle by the pacemaker lead may result in tamponade.

NURSING DIAGNOSIS: HIGH RISK FOR INFECTION

Risk Factors
- Surgical incision allowing for entrance of bacteria
- Invasive procedure
- Placement of lead and/or generator

Patient Outcomes
Patient will be free of infection, as evidenced by
- body temperature < 99°F.
- absence of
  - redness at insertion site
  - purulent drainage at insertion site
  - swelling at insertion site
  - increased warmth at incision site
  - increased pain at incision site
- normal white blood cell (WBC) count and differential

Table 17.1 • Malfunctions and Interventions

Malfunction	Causes	Interventions

1. Noncapture (failure to capture) evidenced by a pacer spike without depolarization, either atrial (P wave) or ventricular (QRS)	Increased pacing threshold
	• Fibrosis
	• Electrolyte imbalance
	• Medications
	• Acid-base disorders
	• Ischemic tissue
	Displacement of lead
	Interruption of pacing system
	Loose lead/generator connection
	Lead fracture
	Battery failure
	Catheter perforation
		Temporary
		• Assess patient for signs of decreased cardiac output.
		• Increase milliamperes; may increase up to 20 mA until capture is regained. If ineffective:
		  –Check all connections and tighten if needed.
		  –Turn patient to left side or position where capture is regained.
		  –Replace battery.
		  –Inform physician.
		• If symptomatic, consider medications, cardiopulmonary resuscitation (CPR) and external pacing until cause is isolated.
		• Anticipate lead repositioning or replacement.
		• Watch for signs of diaphramatic pacing and tamponade.
		
		Permanent
		• Assess patient.
		• Turn patient to left side or position where capture is regained.
		• Watch for signs of diaphramatic pacing and tamponade.
		• Inform physician for reprogramming to increase output of generator.
		• Anticipate possible repositioning or replacement of lead/generator.
		• Have atropine and external pacer available if needed.

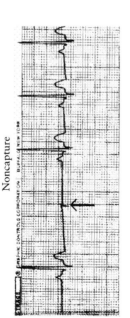

Noncapture

2. Undersensing (nonsensing): evidenced by pacer spikes falling closer to the intrinsic beat than the escape interval (escape interval: see Table 17.4)

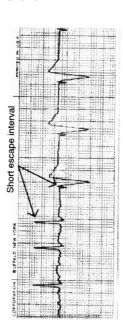

Short escape interval

Inadequate cardiac signal (P wave or R wave).
Interruption in sensing circuit.
- Broken lead
- Lead malpositioned
- Battery failure
- Loose connections

Electromagnetic interference (EMI) which may cause the pacer to revert to asynchonous mode.

EMI: radiated or conducted energy, either electrical or magnetic

Temporary
- Check ECG to make sure intrinsic beats are not within refractory period.
- Check generator to make sure it is not in asynchronous mode.
- Turn patient to position where sensing last seen.
- Increase sensitivity capabilities by turning sensitivity clockwise toward demand mode.
- Tighten all connections.
- Replace battery.
- Notify physician.
- Anticipate lead repositioning or replacement.
- Remove all potential sources of EMI such as an electrical razor.

Permanent
- Assess patient.
- Check ECG to make sure intrinsic beats are not within refractory period.
- Check to make sure there is not a magnet near the pulse generator; magnets over pulse generators will make them asynchronous.
- Turn patient to position where sensing is last seen.
- Inform physician for reprogramming of sensitivity.
- Anticipate possible repositioning or replacement lead/generator.

Table 17.1 • Continued

Malfunction	Causes	Interventions
3. Nonfiring (failure to Fire): evidenced by pauses on ECG tracing longer than automatic interval of pacemaker. Lack of pacer spike at end of escape or automatic interval (automatic interval: see Table 17.4)	Interruption in pacing system. • Loose lead/generator • Connection • Lead failure • Battery failure Over-sensing Inappropriately sensing myopotentials; sensitivity set too high Myopotentials: electrical signals that originate in body muscles. EMI Electrocautery that will inhibit pacing	*Temporary* • Assess patient for signs of decreased cardiac output. • Check all connections and tighten. • Change battery. • Convert pacemaker to asynchronous mode. If pacer spikes return, the pacemaker is able to fire and oversensing is the problem. • Make pacer less sensitive by turning sensitivity counterclockwise toward asynchronous mode. • Check for sources of EMI in room and remove. *Permanent* • Assess patient for signs and symptoms of decreased cardiac output. • If symptomatic, prepare to treat with atropine, external pacemaker, or CPR. • Notify physician for reprogramming of sensitivity if nonfiring is from oversensing. • Anticipate need for lead and/or generator replacement. • Arrange to have pacemaker programmed to asynchronous mode for electrocautery.

Failure to Fire

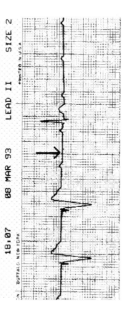

Table 17.2 • Pacer Coding System

The NBG Pacer Code (Five-Letter Code)

1. First letter chamber paced
   a. V = ventricle
   b. A = atrium
   c. D = dual (V & A)
   d. O = none

2. Second letter chamber sensed
   a. V = ventricle
   b. A = atrium
   c. D = dual (V & A)
   d. O = none

3. Third letter mode of response
   a. I = inhibited
   b. T = triggered
   c. D = dual (I & T)
   d. O= none

4. Fourth letter: programmability and rate modulation
   a. O= none
   b. P = simple
   c. M = multiprogrammable
   d. C = communicating
   e. R = rate modulation

5. Fifth letter: antitachyarrhythmia functions
   a. O=none
   b. P = pacing
   c. S = scanning/shock
   d. D = dual

Note: Adapted from "The NASPE/BPEG Generic Pacemaker Code for Antibradyarrhythmia and Adaptive—Rate Pacing and Antitachyarrhythmia Devices" by A. D. Bernstein et al., 1987, *PACE, 10*, 794.

▼

Table 17.3 • Pacing Modes and Descriptions

Mode	Description
AAI	Atrial paced: atrial sensed and inhibited in response to atrial sensing
VVI	Ventricular paced: ventricular sensed and inhibited in response to ventricular sensing
VVIR	Ventricular paced: ventricular sensed and inhibited in response to ventricular sensing Rate responsive
DVI	Atrioventricular (AV) sequential pacing Atrial and ventricular pacing Ventricular sensed Inhibited atrial and ventricular response to ventricular sensing
DDD	Atrial and ventricular pacing Atrial and ventricular sensing Inhibited atrial and ventricular response to atrial and ventricular sensing Triggered ventricular response to atrial sensing
DDDR	Atrial and ventricular pacing Atrial and ventricular sensing Inhibited atrial and ventricular response to atrial and ventricular sensing Triggered ventricular response to atrial sensing Rate responsive

Note: These are some of the common pacing modes. If there is not rate responsiveness, generally only three letters are used. If there is rate responsiveness, four letters are used. If there are antitachycardia functions, five letters are use.

Table 17.4 • Pacing Intervals

Single Chamber

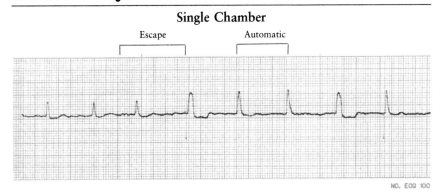

Escape interval: distance between patient's own beat (intrinsic beat) and the next paced beat.

Automatic interval: distance between two consecutive pacing spikes:
1. Equals set rate of pacer
2. V-V interval in ventricular pacing (distance between two consecutive ventricular pacing spikes)
3. A-A interval in atrial pacing (distance between two consecutive atrial pacing spikes)

Dual Chamber: Lower Rate 70 bpm

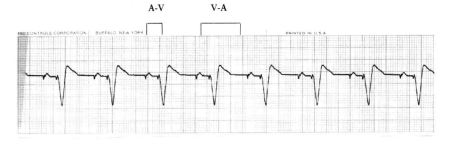

A-V interval: set interval from atrial spike to ventricular spike

V-A interval: atrial escape interval—time from ventricular spike to next atrial spike

V-V interval: lower rate of pacer in milliseconds (ms)

$$\text{Conversion bpm} \quad \text{ms} \quad \frac{60,000 \text{ ms}}{\text{bpm}} \quad \frac{60,000 \text{ ms}}{60 \text{ bpm}} = 1,000 \text{ ms}$$

V-V interval	Example: V-V 60 bpm = 1,000 ms
−A-V interval	A-V interval = −250 ms
V-A interval	V-A interval = 750 ms

Nursing Interventions	Rationales
Monitor temperature every 4 hr and prn. Record and report temperatures above 99°F.	Temperature elevation is a systemic manifestation of infection and is the first sign of infection if the wound is still dressed.
Assess insertion site for redness, purulent drainage, swelling, and warmth.	Intact skin is the natural barrier against invasion of bacteria. An incision and placement of foreign bodies (lead and generator) allow for entrance of bacteria leading to infection. Redness, purulent drainage, swelling, and warmth are indicative of inflammation.
Assess for subjective symptoms of increased pain or tenderness at insertion site.	Inflammation of site leads to increased pain or tenderness.
Monitor WBCs and differential values and report significant elevations.	Inflammatory process stimulates the release of leukocytes and promotes bone marrow production resulting in leukocytosis.
Utilize proper incisional care by 1. maintaining a dry clean occlusive dressing for first 24 hr. 2. changing dressing as ordered or prn if it becomes soiled after first 24 hr. 3. using aseptic technique when changing dressing. 4. keeping incision site dry and clean after dressing discontinued. 5. using strict handwashing techniques for dressing changes. 6. using gloves for removing soiled dressing.	A dry occlusive dressing will absorb drainage, prevent bleeding, and prevent contamination from external sources. Soiled moist dressings are an excellent source of bacterial growth. Aseptic technique and thorough handwashing prevent cross-contamination. Gloves will prevent contact with patient's body fluids.
Administer prophylactic antibiotics as prescribed	Even with strict aseptic technique during insertion and with dressing changes, normal skin flora may cause inflammation and infection at the site.

NURSING DIAGNOSIS: IMPAIRED PHYSICAL MOBILITY

Related To imposed activity restriction and pain at insertion site

Defining Characteristics

Restriction of movement due to mechanical device
Limited range of motion
Restricted movement of arm above shoulder

Patient Outcomes

Permanent Pacemaker
- Able to perform active range of motion of affected site after 48 hr.
- Able to raise arms over head after 5 days
- Absence of a frozen shoulder characterized by joint stiffness, pain, and muscle weakness of extremity.

Temporary Pacemaker
- Participates in passive range-of-motion exercises while pacemaker in place
- Perform active range-of-motion exercises of extremity after pacemaker removed

Nursing Interventions	Rationales
Assess for complications of immobility such as muscle weakness and restricted joint mobility.	Use of muscles and movement promote physical mobility.
Implement measures to prevent complications of immobility, such as: 1. Instruct in range-of-motion exercises. 2. Instruct in isometric exercises of lower extremities. 3. Assist in frequent positional changes. 4. Assist in use of affected extremity 48 hr postimplant (if permanent pacer).	
Offer pain medication prior to use of extremity.	Relief of pain will promote movement of affected area.

NURSING DIAGNOSIS: HIGH RISK FOR IMPAIRED GAS EXCHANGE

Risk Factors
- Percutaneous insertion of lead into intrathoracic vein
- Activity restrictions

Patient Outcomes
Patient will have adequate gas exchange, as evidenced by
- no complaints of SOB
- normal PaO_2 or pulse oximetry
- normal breath sounds throughout lung fields
- Normal chest x-ray without signs of pneumothorax
- no complaints of chest pain

Nursing Interventions	Rationales
Monitor patient for signs and symptoms of pneumothorax, including SOB, chest pain, decreased PaO_2, absence of breath sounds over affected lung, chest x-ray showing pneumothorax	Patient may develop pneumothorax after percutaneous subclavian pacemaker insertion.
Encourage coughing and deep breathing while on bedrest.	Lung expansion will prevent atelectasis.
Assist with changing positions in bed.	Movement improves lung expansion.

NURSING DIAGNOSIS: HIGH RISK FOR IMPAIRED SKIN INTEGRITY

Risk Factors
- Large surface electrodes in transcutaneous pacing
- Immobility
- Elderly

Patient Outcomes
- Patient's skin will remain intact
- No signs of skin trauma (i.e., abrasions, burns) will be noted.

Nursing Interventions	Rationales
Assess skin prior to placement of transcutaneous patches.	
Prepare skin for transcutaneous patches by 1. Cleaning and drying. Do not use alcohol, benzoine, or lotion. 2. Clipping excessive hair. DO NOT SHAVE.	Clean, dry skin will achieve good skin contact, preventing burns. Alcohol, benzoine, and lotions alter skin resistance and increase risk of irritation. Shaving hair may cause abrasions.
Assess skin around pacing electrodes daily for breakdown or burns.	
Reposition and replace electrodes as needed and apply topical burn cream if needed.	Patches cause tissue irritation.
Assist with shifting position frequently. Offer frequent back rubs and massage bony prominences.	

NURSING DIAGNOSIS: KNOWLEDGE DEFICIT

Related To recent diagnosis and lack of readiness to learn about pacemakers

Defining Characteristics
Anxiety over pacer insertion and life-style changes
Lack of recall
Verbalization indicating inadequate understanding of pacemaker concepts and self-care

Patient Outcomes
Patient will verbalize an understanding of
- reason for pacemaker insertion
- insertion procedure
- type of activity restrictions postprocedure
- basic function of the pacemaker
- rationale for continued follow-up
- signs and symptoms of pacemaker malfunction
- facts about electromagnetic interference (see Table 17.5)
- signs and symptoms of infection
Patient will accurately demonstrate how to
- care for pacemaker incision site
- take own pulse

Table 17.5 • Electromagnetic Sources

Static Electricity
Cautery
Defibrillation
Nuclear magnetic resonance
Lithotripsy
Radiation therapy
Magnetic fields
Large electrical cables
Welding currents
All line-powered appliances (shaver, tools, hair blower) are safe unless
   placed directly over pacer and turned off and on repeatedly or if not
   in proper working order.
Spark-ignited engines are safe if properly used.
Radiotransmitters are safe if within guidelines of FCC.
Metal detectors such as airport security are safe but may cause alarm.

Note: Electromagnetic interference (EMI) may inhibit or trigger pacing. If patients
become lightheaded or dizzy when in contact with EMI, they should move away
to see if symptoms resolve. Pacemaker should be checked for possible
reprogramming.

Nursing Interventions	Rationales
Assess readiness to learn and educational needs.	
Assess anxiety level and offer relaxation techniques.	Decreased anxiety will decrease need for sedation and enhance learning ability.
Assess life-style.	Some jobs may involve work with or near magnetic fields, which cause pacemaker interference. Pacemaker sites may be changed from right subclavian area to allow using a gun for hunting or participation in other sports.

Nursing Interventions

Instruct the patient prior to the insertion regarding
1. reason for pacer insertion, including anatomy, physiology, and pathophysiology
2. the procedure (permanent or temporary)
3. site of insertion
4. type of anesthetic to be used
5. type of activity restrictions postprocedure

Instruct using verbal and written information prior to discharge regarding
1. site care
2. activity limitations
3. signs and symptoms of infection
4. signs and symptoms of malfunction
   - weakness
   - dizziness
   - lightheadedness
   - pulse rate lower than low rate of pacemaker
   - loss of consciousness
   - rapid heart rate that does not subside with rest
5. counting of pulse for 1 full minute
6. rationale for pacemaker follow-up
7. facts about electromagnetic interference

Rationales

Thorough instruction and understanding prior to procedure will help alleviate fear of unknown.

Thorough teaching will decrease anxiety about the pacemaker and increase compliance with follow-up.

DISCHARGE PLANNING/CONTINUITY OF CARE

- Provide proper teaching regarding the pacemaker and follow-up.
- Schedule follow-up visit with physician.
- Arrange for instruction in use of transtelephonic monitor if follow-up will be by this method.
- Provide instructions on home medications.

- Instruct on who to call for possible malfunctions or when adverse effects from pacemaker are noted.

REFERENCES

Bernstein, A. D., Camm, A. J., Fletcher, R. D., Gold, R. D., Rickard, A. F., Smyth, N. P., Spielman, S. R., & Sutton, R. (1987). The NASPE/BPEG generic code for antibradyarrhythmia and adaptive-rate pacing and antitachyarrhythmia devices. *PACE, 10,* 794.

Guzzetta, C. E., & Montgomery Dossey, B. (1992). *Cardiovascular nursing: Holistic practice.* St. Louis, MO: Mosby Year Book.

Kinney, M. R., Packa, D. R., Andreoli, K. G., & Zipes, D. P. (1991). *Comprehensive cardiac case* (7th ed.). St. Louis, MO: Mosby Year Book.

Montgomery Dossey, B., Guzzetta, C. E., & Vanderstaay Kenner, C. (1992). *Critical care nursing: Body-mind-spirit.* Philadelphia: Lippincott Company.

Moses, H., Schneider, J., Miller, B., & Taylor, G. (1991). *A practical guide to cardiac pacing* (3rd ed.). Boston: Little, Brown.

Tiputz, L. (1991). Cardiac pacemakers. *Journal of Cardiovascular Nursing, 5*(3), 1–85.

Underhil, S., Woods, S., Froelicher, E., & Halpenny C. (1989). *Cardiac nursing* (2nd ed.). Philadelphia: Lippincott.

▼

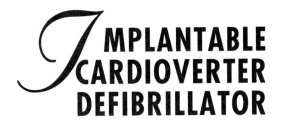

IMPLANTABLE CARDIOVERTER DEFIBRILLATOR

Cherri A. Schleicher, RN, BSN, CCRN

The implantable cardioverter defibrillator (ICD) is an internally implanted device designed to monitor the heart rhythm. If the ICD detects ventricular tachycardia or ventricular fibrillation, it automatically delivers an electric impulse to the heart to return it to normal sinus rhythm. Depending on the type of device implanted, this impulse may consist of small rapid pacing pulses or a larger electric countershock. Some of the newer devices also include bradycardia pacing as well as antitachycardia pacing.

An ICD is indiceed for patients at risk of sudden cardiac death from ventricular tachycardia or fibrillation. The device is implanted surgically under a general anesthetic. The surgical approach depends on the type of device implanted and if any concomitant surgery is being done. The types of approaches used in implanting the ICD include sternotomy, thoracotomy, the subxyphoid approach, and transvenous and submuscular insertions.

Sternotomy is used most often when other surgery such as coronary artery bypass grafting is done in conjunction with the ICD. The main incision is made lengthwise over the breastbone, with a small incision in the left upper abdomen for implantation of the generator.

Thoracotomy may be chosen for a person who has already had chest surgery or who may have scar tissue around the heart. The main incision is made between the ribs on the left side; a small incision is made in the upper abdomen for the generator.

Transvenous nonthoracotomy is the newest of the surgical approaches available and it is least invasive. With the transvenous insertion a small incision is made near the collarbone, and a lead is threaded through a vein to the heart. The tip of the lead lies in the right ventricle. A small incision is made on the left chest wall at the fifth or sixth intercostal space. A patch is placed just under the skin on top of the ribs. A small incision will also be made in the abdomen for the generator.

In the subxiphoid approach the main insicion is made lengthwise below and slightly to the left of the breastbone, along with the generator incision. Used also as an alternative to thoracotomy.

ETIOLOGIES

Ventricular tachycardia/fibrillation
- Coronary artery disease with ischemia or infarction
- Cardiomyopathy–ischemic/congestive/idiopathic
- Primary electrical disease–prolonged QT syndrome
- Valvular heart disease

CLINICAL MANIFESTATIONS

Ventricular tachycardia/fibrillation
- Sudden death
- Syncope
- Palpitations
- Breathlessness
- Hypotension
- Dizziness/lightheadedness
- Chest pain/angina

CLINICAL/DIAGNOSTIC FINDINGS

Noninvasive tests
- Electrocardiography
  - ventricular ectopy and left ventricular enlargement
  - ischemia
  - aneurysm formation
  - infarction
- Signal-average electrocardiography
  Reveals late potentials. These are signals that are depicted on an electrocardiogram (ECG) and are associated with a greater potential for ventricular tachycardia or fibrillation.
- Holter monitor
  - ventricular ectopy
- Echocardiography
  - left ventricular hypertrophy
  - left ventricular free wall motion abnormalities
  - akinesis, hypokinesis of ventricles
  - decreased left ventricular ejection fraction
  - valvular insufficiency or stenosis
- Multigated blood imaging (MUGA) scan
  - wall motion abnormalities
  - decreased right ventricular ejection fraction
  - decreased left ventricular ejection fraction

Invasive tests
- Electrophysiology study
  - determines inducibility of ventricular tachycardia or fibrillation and physiological tolerance of dysrhythmia

NURSING DIAGNOSIS: HIGH RISK FOR DECREASED CARDIAC OUTPUT

Risk Factors
- Implantation of ICD
- Life-threatening ventricular dysrhythmias
- Variations in blood pressure
- Syncope

Patient Outcomes
- Cardiac output will be maintained, as evidenced by:
  - regular pulse or heart rate 60–100
  - normal blood pressure
  - no complaints of syncope
  - no complaints of shortness of breath
  - warm, dry skin
- Life-threatening arrhythmias will be detected, effectively treated, and reported.

Nursing Interventions	Rationales
Note on patient's record the on/off status of the ICD.	This is essential to evaluate functioning of the device.
Monitor the ECG.	Continuous monitoring is necessary to detect dysrhythmia and evaluate ICD function.
Allow a specified amount of time for the ICD to identify dysrhythmia and start to charge and discharge, according to the ICD device.	Normally, the ICD does not discharge until a certain number of ventricular beats are detected. This is dependent on device type and programmed options. It is essential to have this recorded on patient's record.
Prepare to defibrillate patient externally and carry out immediately if device is turned off or not functioning.	A patient can be externally defibrillated with an ICD. The anterior-posterior position is preferable, but the anterior-anterior paddle position may also be used.

Nursing Interventions	Rationales
Document ICD discharge on ECG rhythm strip.	This is necessary to evaluate appropriate ICD function.
Monitor and document blood pressure and sensorium during and after ventricular tachycardia/fibrillation.	In a rapid tachycardia the cardiac output can be compromised and a decrease in blood pressure and level of consciousness will occur.
Begin antidysrhythmic medication as prescribed.	Intravenous (IV) lidocaine or other agents may be necessary to minimize further dysrhythmias.
If life-threatening rhythm is converted, notify physician and continue to monitor closely for hemodynamic compromise.	Decrease in blood pressure and increase in pulse rate may occur as a result of dysrhythmia and medications administered.
If life-threatening rhythm remains, start resuscitative measures according to hospital procedures.	Further hemodynamic deterioration may occur following defibrillation, requiring emergency measures.

NURSING DIAGNOSIS: ACUTE PAIN

Related To recent incisional or muscular discomfort from surgery

Defining Characteristics
Muscle discomfort
Tissue trauma
Restlessness, agitation, or anxiety

Patient Outcomes
Patient will be free of pain, as evidenced by
- verbal expression of relief of pain
- stable blood pressure and pulse rate
- decrease in restlessness or anxiety
- ability to resume normal activities

Nursing Interventions	Rationales
Assess the patient's pain and characteristics of the pain by asking the location, intensity, and duration. Having the patient rate the pain on a scale of–10.	Surgical pain needs to be differentiated from anginal pain, as treatment will be different.

Nursing Interventions	Rationales
Monitor blood pressure, pulse, and respiratory rate during pain and after pain relief.	The most common physiological changes indicative of acute pain are changes in blood pressure, pulse, and respirations.
Implement nonpharmacological interventions that assist in controlling pain, that is, behavioral approaches and guided imagery.	Nonpharmacological pain control measures optimize pharmacological agents and promote comfort.
Provide adequate rest periods.	Pain can be intensified by fatigue.
Administer analgesics 30 min prior to any invasive test or activity.	Analgesics decrease pain, allowing the patient to slowly resume normal activity.
Evaluate effectiveness of pain control measures.	
Support and guide the patient in making decisions regarding pain control measures.	Patient preferences are important in achieving effective pain control measures.

NURSING DIAGNOSIS: HIGH RISK FOR INFECTION

Risk Factors
- Disruption of skin surfaces
- Invasion of body surfaces

Patient Outcomes
- Patient will be free of infection, as evidenced by
  - normal wound healing
  - white blood cell (WBC) count 5,000–10,000 with normal differential
  - no infiltrate on chest x-ray (CXR)
  - no chills or cough
  - body temperature < 100°F
- Febrile state will be detected and controlled.

Nursing Interventions	Rationales
Assess skin integrity and incisions, observing for any redness, tenderness, or warmth.	The first sign of infection may be erythema, tenderness, or swelling at the site.

Nursing Interventions	Rationales
Monitor WBC count, temperature, and respirations. Note any cough and infiltrate on CXR.	Common sites of postoperative infection are the lungs and upper respiratory tract.
Maintain good hand-washing technique.	Good hand washing is the most important strategy to prevent infections.
Clean incisions according to prescribed protocol.	Aseptic technique prevents infection.
Insert indwelling lines and tubes under sterile conditions and maintain aseptically.	Skin is the first line of defense against infection.

NURSING DIAGNOSIS: IMPAIRED ADJUSTMENT

Related To
- Change in body image
- Change in self-esteem
- Change in roles
- Change in financial status
- Inadequate support systems

Defining Characteristics
Change in appearance of chest and abdomen
Outline of defibrillator visible, particularily in thin people
Verbalizations such as "I don't feel comfortable wearing tight-fitting clothes" and "I feel everyone can see the outline of my defibrillator"
Lack of movement toward independence

Patient Outcomes
- The patient will participate in normal activities.
- Patient and family financial concerns will be addressed.
- Fears, concerns, and expectations will be verbalized.

Nursing Interventions	Rationales
Allow time for patient/family to express feelings and concerns.	A high level of patient and family stress is associated with ventricular dysrhythmia.
Assist patient and family with contacting insurance company to ascertain coverage of the ICD.	Financial concerns contribute to overall stress, and most patients can be assured that ICD implantation is a covered procedure.

Nursing Interventions	Rationales
Contact department of social services or financial counseling as appropriate.	When financial concerns arise, services can be provided to assist with individual financial planning.
Allow verbalization of feelings regarding appearance.	Most patients will have surgical incisions on their chest and upper abdomen plus a generator under the skin which measures approximately $\frac{1}{2} \times 2\frac{1}{2} \times 3\frac{1}{2}$ inches.
Encourage looking at and touching insertion site.	In addition to promoting acceptance of the device, this gives the patient a baseline for detection of future problems.
Encourage wearing own clothing; suggest abdominal binder for comfort.	Abdominal binder gives added support and in turn will give comfort.
Promote the lifesaving nature of the device.	Acceptance is enhanced by the realization of the necessity of the device.
Have person with an ICD visit patient and family.	Hearing from a patient's point of view that life can be quite normal after ICD implantation is helpful and reassuring to patients.
Encourage patient/family participation in support groups.	Observation, exploration of feelings, and perceptions are important assessment strategies.
Review activity limitations, such as lifting restrictions, when appropriate to life-style.	Knowledge of specific limitations will encourage patient participation in normal activity and decrease anxiety.

NURSING DIAGNOSIS: SLEEP PATTERN DISTURBANCE

Related To
- Effects of medication
- Change in activity patterns
- Fear of malfunction of ICD device
- Fear of frequent shocks and what ICD shock feels like
- Change in roles/life-style
- Change in sleep routine

Defining Characteristics

Awakening early and not being able to go back to sleep
Fatigue
Expressionless face
Dark circles under eyes
Inability to concentrate

Patient Outcomes

- Factors that contribute to sleep pattern disturbance and factors that promote an optimal sleep pattern will be described.
- An optimal balance between sleep and activity will be demonstrated.
- Increased satisfaction with sleep pattern will be verbalized.

Nursing Interventions	Rationales
Explore the physiological, psychological, and environmental factors that may be interfering with sleep.	The hospital environment can be noisy and the transition to home stressful, affecting sleep patterns. Incisional discomfort and fear of device firing also compound the problem.
Assess present sleep and activity patterns.	A detailed assessment is necessary before appropriate intervention can be planned.
Assess the effects of medications on the sleep patterns.	A review of the medication profile may reveal medications which interfere with sleep patterns.
Discuss relaxation and other sleep-promoting techniques that are appropriate (e.g., imagery, progressive muscle relaxation, positive thinking, exercise, maintaining regular sleep hours).	Daily personal routines and patient preference are important in relaxation techniques.

NURSING DIAGNOSIS: KNOWLEDGE DEFICIT

Related To complex treatment plan

Defining Characteristics

Verbalization indicating inadequate understanding of or inability to perform desired health behaviors.

Patient Outcomes

The patient and family will verbalize understanding of
- device need and function
- self-care and resumption of normal acitivities
- signs and symptoms of infection
- electrical or magnetic interferences with the device
- medical identification
- medications and their side effects
- what to do if the ICD discharges
- follow-up care

Nursing Interventions	Rationales
Assess baseline knowledge.	Educational, cultural, and social backgrounds influence knowledge base.
Provide written materials such as booklets and pamphlets on the ICD.	There are teaching booklets available from the companies that make the device or from dysrhythmia clinics.
Allow time to review materials and provide individualized teaching with patient and family.	Verbally reviewing information and allowing time for questions help to assess understanding and individualize information.
Discuss ICD cut-off rate and when ICD will discharge.	Knowledge of ICD cut-off rate will help the patient to monitor his or her own activity. A typical cut-off rate is 160, and patients need to understand that they should avoid activities that would increase the heart rate above this level.
Discuss ICD electromagnetic interferences, such as stereo speakers, airport security wands, industrial equipment, arc welders, large generators, and power plants.	It is important for a patient to avoid contact with strong magnetic fields. In previous models (Ventak 1550/1600) contact with a magnetic field deactivated the ICD. Newer models (Medtronic PCD) are inhibited by magnetic fields but are not deactivated.
Discuss medication, dosages, purpose, and side effects.	Knowing the dosage and purpose of the medication increases knowledge and promotes compliance. Knowing the side effects can prevent complications and toxic effects from medications.

Nursing Interventions	Rationales
Provide medication teaching sheets and self-care information sheets.	Providing written material is a valuable resource for patients and families in understanding their care.
Teach the importance of emergency numbers and medic alert information.	Family members should be taught to call their emergency facility in the event of multiple shocks from the defibrillator or if the patient collapses. Medic alert jewelry is important so other health care professionals can identify the type of defibrillator patient has.
Encourage family members, if appropriate (depending on age and health status), to learn cardiopulmonary resuscitation (CPR).	Prompt and effective CPR can increase patient survival by 30–40%.

DISCHARGE PLANNING/CONTINUITY OF CARE

- Ensure that patient/family know ICD cut-off rate and settings and are aware that exceeding the cut-off rate can cause the device to discharge.
- Inform patients who have had transvenous systems placed or nonthoracotomy systems that they are restricted in lifting the left arm above shoulder level for 4–6 weeks after surgery, so as not to dislodge the lead. Routine dressing/writing are not contraindicated. Encourage gradual increase in activity or involvement in a cardiac rehabilitation program.
- Give patient a medic alert identification card on discharge stating own name and address and model and serial number of the ICD as well as physician name. The patient should be encouraged to order medic alert jewelry.
- Inform patient that prior to any surgical procedure the ICD must be deactivated and prior to any surgical or dental procedure antibiotics are prescribed to prevent infection from occurring on the leads, patches, or generator site. Patients or their physician should call the electrophysiologist prior to performing the procedure.
- Give a list of out-of-state/country centers which can assist in the event of ICD malfunctioning. Advise patient that the ICD can cause an airport metal detector alarm to go off. Airport personnel should be shown an ICD identification card. Airport wands have a strong magnetic field and can potentially interfere with the device, so they should not be used.

- Inform patient that electromagnetic interferences can be caused by close contact with a strong magnetic field (such as the antena of a CB radio, the alternator of a running car, or a large transformer) and that such contact should be avoided when possible.
- Emphasize the importance of follow-up for ICD care.

REFERENCES

Keren, R., Aarons, D., & Veltri, E.(1991). Anxiety and depression in patients with life-threatening ventricular arrhythmias; Impact of the implantable cardioverter defibrillator. *PACE, 14,* 181–186.

Kupier, R. A. (1990). The automatic implantable cardioverter defibrillator as a therapeutic modality for recurrent ventricular tachycardia. A case study. *Progress in Cardiovascular Nursing, 5*(1), 6–11.

McFarlane, E. A., & McFarlane, G. K. (1989). *Nursing diagnosis and intervention, planning for patient care.* St. Louis, MO: Mosby.

Noel, D. K., Burke, L. J., Martinez, B., Petrie, K., Stack, T., & Cudworth, K. L. (1986). Challenging concerns for patient with automatic implantable cardioverter defibrillator. *Focus on Critical Care, 13*(6), 50–57.

Teplitz, L., Egenes, K. J., & Brask, L. (1990). Life after sudden death; the development of a support group for automatic implantable cardioverter defibrillator patients. *Journal of Cardiovascular Nursing, 4*(2), 20–33.

Veseth-Rogers, J. (1990). A practical approach to teaching the automatic implantable cardioverter defibrillator patient. *Journal of Cardiovascular Nursing, 4*(2), 7–19.

▼

$\mathcal{V}$ENTRICULAR ASSIST DEVICE

Claire C. Elsesser, RN, BSN, CCRN

Ventricular assist devices (VADs) provide temporary circulatory support for patients with ventricular failure. A VAD diverts blood flow around a failing ventricle by using surgically or percutaneously placed cannulae and an external or implanted blood pump. A right or left ventricular assist device (RVAD or LVAD) may be used to support a single ventricle that has failed or bi-ventricular support (Bi-VAD) may be indicated. Cannulae are placed in the right atrium or ventricle and the pulmonary artery to bypass the right ventricle. Likewise, cannulae are placed in the left atrium or ventricle and the aorta to bypass the left ventricle. The cannulae are connected to the blood pump. A driveline extends from the blood pump to the VAD console, which controls pumping.

The intra-aortic balloon pump (IABP) is the simplest and most commonly used form of VAD support, although several other types of VADs are available for patients with profound cardiac failure who do not respond to an IABP. These devices provide partial or complete support and are used to stabilize patients until myocardial recovery is achieved or cardiac transplantation is performed. Some of these devices are FDA approved (e.g., Medtronics-Biomedicus, Abiomed, Bard Cardiopulmonary Support System), but many are part of investigational clinical trials (e.g., Thoratec, Thermo Cardiosystems Inc. HeartMate, Novacor). Some VADs are prototypes for long-term support, and in the future may be used in place of cardiac transplantation.

ETIOLOGIES

- Right and/or left ventricular failure
- Postcardiotomy ventricular failure
- Cardiogenic shock following myocardial infarction
- End-stage cardiomyopathy
- Failure of a transplanted heart

268

CLINICAL MANIFESTATIONS

- Signs of progressive ventricular failure despite pharmacological and/or IABP therapy
- Hemodynamic criteria for initiating VAD support
  - cardiac index (CI) < 2 L/min/m^2
  - systolic blood pressure (SBP) < 90 mmHg or mean arterial pressure (MAP) < 60 mmHg
  - left and/or right atrial pressure (LAP/RAP) > 20 mmHg
  - systemic vascular resistance (SVR) > 2100 dyn/s/cm^{-5}
  - urine output < 20 mL/hr
- Decreased level of consciousness
- Respiratory compromise requiring ventilatory support
- Pulmonary edema

CLINICAL/DIAGNOSTIC FINDINGS

- Electrocardiogram (ECG) findings
  - tachycardia
  - premature atrial or ventricular contractions
  - ventricular tachycardia or fibrillation
  - evidence of infarction
- Chest x-ray
  - cardiomegaly
  - pulmonary vascular engorgement
  - alveolar or interstitial edema
- Echocardiography
  - decreased ejection fraction
  - hypokinesis/akinesis
- Cardiac catheterization: coronary artery occlusion

NURSING DIAGNOSIS: DECREASED CARDIAC OUTPUT

Related To decreased vascular volume, increased afterload, dysrhythmias, and/or VAD malfunction.

Defining Characteristics
Decreased VAD output
Decreased MAP
Decreased RAP, LAP/pulmonary capillary wedge pressure (PCWP)
Decreased cardiac output/index (CO/CI)
Increased SVR, pulmonary vascular resistance (PVR)
Dysrhythmias
Signs of bleeding

Patient Outcomes

Patient will

- maintain adequate CO on VAD support as evidenced by VAD output 2–5 L/min with improved CI and normal MAP, RAP, LAP/PCWP, SVR, and PVR.
- be free of dysrhythmias that affect VAD output.
- maintain hematological function, as evidenced by control of bleeding and coagulation studies within prescribed parameters.

Nursing Interventions	Rationales
Assess LVAD and/or RVAD console function continuously and document VAD parameters on flowsheet hourly [e.g., VAD output, mode, VAD rate, systolic duration, stroke volume, drive pressure(s), vacuum].	The VAD can maintain partial or complete circulatory flow. Changes in VAD parameters require immediate patient assessment to determine probable cause, appropriate medical or mechanical intervention, and maintenance of VAD output.
Assess trends in hemodynamic pressures (MAP, RAP, LAP/PCWP). (See Table 5.1 for normal hemodynamic values.)	Adequate atrial pressure and volume must be maintained to achieve VAD filling and optimal VAD output.
Evaluate thermodilution CO in LVAD patients only. Assess trends in hemodynamic profile. The VAD output may be used for calculation of hemodynamic profile in RVAD or Bi-VAD patients.	Thermodilution CO is inaccurate in patients with an RVAD or Bi-VAD because blood flow through the RVAD affects the temperature and flow of the blood.
Assess MAP, SVR, and PVR.	The VAD output will be decreased in the presence of increased afterload. Elevated MAP, SVR, and/or PVR require the use of afterload-reducing drugs.

Nursing Interventions	Rationales
Monitor heart rate and rhythm: 1. Institute standard antidysrhythmic therapy when dysrhythmia affects VAD output. 2. Defibrillate prn for ventricular tachycardia or fibrillation unless on a Bi-VAD. 3. Avoid cardiopulmonary resuscitation (CPR) whenever possible. Call physician to perform open chest cardiac massage if indicated. Perform closed chest compressions only as a final option.	A Bi-VAD will function and maintain adequate CO despite lethal dysrhythmias. Persistent ventricular tachycardia or fibrillation may be treated more aggressively in patients expected to recover ventricular function versus those awaiting transplant. In the presence of a single RVAD or LVAD, dysrhythmias require immediate treatment. Caution must be used when defibrillating in the presence of a VAD or cannulae with metal components. Arcing may occur. Special defibrillation skin pads are recommended.
Assess for failure of the unassisted ventricle in LVAD or RVAD patients and notify the physician promptly. Right ventricular failure with an LVAD will cause increased RAP, poor LVAD filling, and decreased LVAD output. Left ventricular failure with an RVAD will cause increased LAP/PCWP with pulmonary edema.	Prompt intervention may prevent the need for Bi-VAD support.
Titrate inotropic and vasoactive infusions for desired effects (e.g., dopamine, dobutamine, nitroprusside, isoproterenol, prostaglandin E_1). (See Tables 5.3 and 5.4 for more information on vasoactive drugs.)	These pharmacological agents are used to enhance contractility of the native heart and to reduce ventricular afterload.
Position patient and VAD to achieve optimal VAD filling. Patient position should be varied according to tolerance. Prevent kinks in cannulae or driveline(s). Support external VAD(s) on abdomen.	The VAD may not fill properly with change in position. Kinks in inflow or outflow cannulae or driveline(s) will affect VAD output.

Nursing Interventions	Rationales
Based on clinical status, adjust VAD mode, rate, systolic duration, drive pressure(s), and/or vacuum as needed to achieve desired VAD output. 1. Consult with technical support staff and/or physician prn. 2. Correct underlying patient problem before adjusting VAD settings. Temporary VAD adjustments may be necessary until volume or afterload status is corrected.	
Document significant patient events or console alarms/problems and interventions on VAD flowsheet. Notify physician prn.	
Detect signs of bleeding: 1. Assess hourly chest tube drainage. 2. Observe incisional, intravenous, cannula, and driveline sites for bleeding. 3. Assess for presence of petechiae, ecchymosis, or blood in body secretions. 4. Evaluate chest x-ray for hemothorax. 5. Monitor complete blood count, coagulation studies, and plasma hemoglobin.	Bleeding is a common complication. Factors that increase the risk of bleeding include prolonged cardiopulmonary bypass, VAD design and synthetic materials, use of high drive pressures or vacuum, impaired liver function, and anticoagulation therapy.
Report evidence of bleeding to physician: 1. Replace blood products. Autotransfuse in acute post-VAD recovery period when appropriate. 2. Use white cell filters when administering whole blood and packed red blood cells in pretransplant patients. 3. Prepare for possible return to surgery.	Circulating volume must be restored quickly to maintain VAD output. White cell filters are indicated to reduce antigen exposure and antibody formation, which may increase the risk of posttransplant rejection.

Nursing Interventions	**Rationales**
Follow specific VAD research protocols (e.g., frequency of documenting patient and VAD data, venting, removal of condensation from driveline).	The Federal Drug Administration (FDA) requires manufacturers of investigational devices to specify research protocols, and centers using the devices are responsible for accurate data collection.
Perform and document a VAD safety check every 8 hr (e.g., battery charge indicators, security of driveline connections, back-up console at bedside when applicable, manual back-up procedures accessible).	Routine safety checks may prevent console problems.
Implement device-specific emergency back-up procedures or switch console in the event of console failure. When changing a Bi-VAD console, disconnect and reconnect drivelines as follows: Disconnect right, then left driveline; reconnect left, then right driveline.	Pumping the RVAD without a functional LVAD will cause pulmonary edema.
Initiate VAD weaning as ordered and monitor response.	The VAD may be adjusted to provide complete or partial support. Weaning plans will vary based on recovery status versus bridge to transplant.

NURSING DIAGNOSIS: ALTERED TISSUE PERFUSION

Related To myocardial dysfunction or thromboembolic complications

Defining Characteristics
Decreased CO/CI
Unstable hemodynamic pressures
Decreased mixed venous oxygen saturation (SvO_2)
Altered consciousness and motor function
Weak peripheral pulses
Capillary refill time (CRT) > 3 s
Pale, cool, moist skin
Urine output < 30 mL/hr
Impaired gastrointestinal (GI) function
Pain

Patient Outcomes

- Patient will maintain adequate perfusion of vital body systems, as evidenced by
  - CO $\geq$ 4 L/min
  - CI $\geq$ 2.5 L/min/m^2
  - MAP > 60 mmHg
  - stable hemodynamic pressures
  - SvO$_2$ $\geq$ 60%
  - alert and oriented with normal motor function
  - palpable peripheral pulses
  - CRT < 3 s
  - warm, dry, pink skin
  - urine output > 30 mL/hr
  - normal GI function
- Patient will maintain therapeutic level of anticoagulation.

Nursing Interventions	Rationales
Evaluate trends in MAP, RAP, LAP/PCWP, CO, and CI.	Deterioration of hemodynamic status results in decreased perfusion of body systems and potential multiorgan compromise.
Monitor trends in SvO$_2$ via a pulmonary artery catheter.	Decreased SvO$_2$ may be an early indicator of an imbalance between oxygen supply and demand.
Assess neurological status: level of consciousness, mentation, verbal response, eye signs, movement of extremities, and sensation. Report significant findings to physician and evaluate cause.	Neurological compromise may be related to decreased cerebral perfusion. There is also a risk of thromboembolic complications associated with clot formation in the VAD or native ventricle, especially with low VAD outputs or low-CO states.
Assess skin color, temperature, presence of edema, quality of peripheral pulses, and CRT.	Signs of decreased peripheral perfusion include cool, pale, mottled, and moist extremities, decreased quality of peripheral pulses, and CRT above 3 s.
Evaluate hourly urine output, daily weight, and daily intake and output and monitor daily laboratory values (electrolytes, BUN, creatinine).	Assessment of renal function and fluid balance indicators leads to prompt diagnosis and intervention for renal compromise.

Nursing Interventions	Rationales
Assess GI function: Auscultate bowel sounds, amount and characteristics of GI drainage, abdominal size, abdominal pain, and presence of nausea or vomiting.	Decreased perfusion or intra-abdominal placement of VAD may cause GI dysfunction.
Notify physician regarding early signs of decreased tissue perfusion to body systems.	Decreased perfusion may cause multiorgan compromise.
Assess external VAD for visual presence of fibrin when applicable.	Synthetic biomaterials have improved, but clot formation is a potential problem.
Administer anticoagulation therapy after chest tube drainage has decreased and there is no evidence of bleeding. Protocol may include heparin, warfarin, dextran, dipyridamole, and aspirin.	Anticoagulation therapy reduces the risk of thrombus formation.
Monitor prothrombin time (PT), partial thromboplastin time (PTT), or activated clotting time (ACT) to achieve therapeutic level of anticoagulation.	Frequent determinations of PT, PTT, or ACT are indicated. Activated clotting times may be done at the bedside.
Implement measures to maintain skin integrity (e.g., repositioning, range-of-motion exercises, air mattress, pressure relief devices).	Compromised tissue perfusion, immobility, and prolonged hospitalization may contribute to skin breakdown. Routine repositioning may not be tolerated until hemodynamically stable.
Monitor effectiveness of fluid replacement therapy, avoiding fluid excess or deficit.	Fluctuations in circulatory volume will affect VAD output, myocardial dysfunction, and organ perfusion.
Monitor response to renal support therapy (dialysis or hemofiltration) when indicated.	Dialysis may affect volume status leading to decreased VAD output. Hemofiltration circuit may be affected by low-flow states.

NURSING DIAGNOSIS: HIGH RISK FOR IMPAIRED GAS EXCHANGE

Risk Factors
- Decreased cardiac reserve
- Pulmonary congestion/edema
- Anesthesia
- Cardiopulmonary bypass: prolonged due to complicated surgery and VAD placement
- VAD pump and cannulae placement
- History of lung disease
- Atelectasis
- Pain
- Sedation
- Immobility

Patient Outcomes
Patient will maintain adequate gas exchange, as evidenced by
- ABGs within patient's normal range
- clear breath sounds
- clearing chest x-ray
- effective respiratory pattern
- extubation following stabilization of VAD output
- absence of cyanosis

Nursing Interventions	Rationales
Evaluate ABGs. Monitor oxygen saturation and noninvasive end-tidal CO_2 concentration continuously. Use in-line continuous blood gas monitor if ABG sampling is frequent and prolonged.	Close surveillance is required in the acute post-VAD recovery period. Fluctuations in acid-base balance and oxygenation are typical.
Assess respiratory pattern, lung sounds, and color of nail beds and mucous membranes.	Early detection and intervention for deteriorating ventilation or oxygenation may prevent complications.
Evaluate daily chest x-rays for status of lung fields and position of endotracheal tube.	

Nursing Interventions	**Rationales**
Maintain airway patency: 1. Suction as indicated by lung auscultation. 2. Assess characteristics and amount of secretions. 3. Use in-line suction catheter if excessive secretions.	Secretion management may require frequent suctioning in the acute phase.
Maintain ventilator support: 1. Assess patient synchrony with ventilator. 2. Use analgesics, sedation, and paralyzing agents prn. 3. Maintain and evaluate response to positive end-expiratory pressure (PEEP). 4. Wean and extubate as soon as condition allows.	When hemodynamically stable, early extubation is optimal for patient comfort and to avoid the complications associated with prolonged intubation.
Elevate head of bed, reposition, and gradually progress exercise and activity as tolerated.	Change in position and activity promotes lung expansion.
Implement postextubation pulmonary measures: 1. oxygen and humidity therapy 2. coughing and deep breathing 3. respiratory treatments 4. progressive exercise and activity as tolerated	Preventive measures minimize complications.
Manage pain.	Pain control promotes effective respiratory patterns and increases tolerance of respiratory treatments and activity.

NURSING DIAGNOSIS: IMPAIRED PHYSICAL MOBILITY

Related To
- VAD placement
- Invasive lines and tubes
- Pre-VAD disability
- Pain

Defining Characteristics

Activity intolerance
Decreased joint mobility
Loss of muscle strength
Pain
Skin breakdown

Patient Outcomes

Patient will
• maintain skin integrity.
• maintain muscle strength and joint mobility.
• tolerate activity progression.

Nursing Interventions	Rationales
Assess skin condition.	Compromised peripheral perfusion predisposes to skin breakdown.
Provide skin care. Use air mattress or pressure relief devices.	Prevention of skin breakdown is critical in the acute post-VAD period when activity is most limited.
Reposition as soon as condition allows. Tilt, turn, and position on side. Maintain proper body alignment.	Repositioning prevents skin breakdown and improves ventilation and secretion removal.
Progress activity as tolerated and monitor response: Elevate head of bed, dangle, chair, and ambulate. Medicate for pain as needed.	Begin limited activity while intubated when possible, and progress activity plan after extubation.
Initiate physical therapy activity/exercise program: 1. Progress from passive to active range of motion. 2. Include bedside exercises to increase endurance and muscle strength (e.g., weights, stationary bicycle). 3. Intensify exercise program as tolerated and include in daily schedule. 4. Transport to physical therapy department when applicable.	A planned exercise program will improve physical status in preparation for cardiac transplantation.

Nursing Interventions	Rationales
Protect VAD cannulae/driveline(s) and support external VAD(s) with activity or transport. Prevent tension or kinking.	Potential decreased VAD output, dislodgement, or damage to sensors may occur.
Instruct patient to protect driveline(s) and support VAD(s) during activity when able. Patient may push VAD console during ambulation, if not too cumbersome.	
Assess VAD battery status indicators before and during ambulation or transport. Minimize time on battery and reconnect to power source as soon as possible.	Battery time will vary on different types of VAD consoles.
Encourage participation in activities of daily living (ADLs) as soon as possible. Obtain occupational therapy consult.	Participation in ADLs increases independence and maximizes feelings of control.
Initiate dietary consult and implement appropriate nutritional support. Progress diet as tolerated. Allow selection of food, and encourage family to bring in favorite foods. Monitor daily weight.	Adequate nutritional intake is required to meet metabolic needs during recovery or in preparation for cardiac transplantation.

NURSING DIAGNOSIS: HIGH RISK FOR INFECTION

Risk Factors
- Presence of VAD, cannulae, and driveline(s)
- Invasive lines and tubes
- Surgical procedures
- Immobility
- Compromised immune response related to critical illness
- Impaired nutrition
- Critical care unit environment

Patient Outcomes
Patient will be free of infection, as evidenced by
- temperature < 100 °F.
- clean, dry incisional and invasive line sites
- clean, dry VAD cannula/driveline sites

- normal white blood cell (WBC) and differential counts
- negative cultures

Nursing Interventions	Rationales
Assess and report temperature elevation, local signs of line or incisional infection, evidence of pulmonary or urinary infection, and increased WBC/abnormal differential count.	Ongoing surveillance is critical to detect early signs of infection. The risk of infection is present throughout the recovery period.
Inspect cannula/driveline sites for presence of redness, heat, swelling, pain, and drainage.	Signs of local infection should be treated promptly. Pain may be an early indicator.
Wash hands before and after care. Apply principles of aseptic technique in all nursing care. Follow institutional protocol for degree of protective isolation. Limit number of caregivers in direct contact with patient.	Isolation protocols may vary. In the immediate post-VAD period, mask and hand washing are usually required. Once stable, good hand washing may be adequate.
Provide daily cannulae/driveline site care according to protocol.	Specific research protocols or manufacturer's guidelines must be considered. Betadine and acetone may cause damage to some VAD cannulae.
Follow protocol for invasive line and incisional care. Assess for normal wound healing. Maintain protective sternal covering in the event of an open sternum.	
Discontinue invasive lines and tubes as soon as condition allows. Consider placement of special long-term intravenous catheter when indicated. Keep written record of line insertion dates, and change site of invasive line according to protocol.	Long-term intravenous catheters avoid the trauma of frequent venipunctures to administer medications or draw blood.

Nursing Interventions	Rationales
Administer antibiotics, antipyretics, and hypothermia therapy as prescribed.	Infections are a common complication of VAD surgery but can be treated effectively with appropriate antibiotics, antipyretics, and hypothermia to lower body temperature and reduce metabolic demands.
Culture any suspicious drainage.	Early identification of specific organisms leads to early treatment.
Screen visitors to avoid contact with infected persons. Instruct visitors regarding isolation procedures.	Patients on VADs are at risk of acquired infection, which may compromise the outcome of future surgery to remove the device.

NURSING DIAGNOSIS: HIGH RISK FOR INEFFECTIVE INDIVIDUAL AND/OR FAMILY COPING

Risk Factors
- Critical condition/fear of impending death
- Use of investigational VAD support system
- Knowledge deficit related to VAD and/or transplant
- Pain
- Immobility
- Critical care environment
- Sleep deprivation
- Family separation

Patient Outcomes
Patient and family will
- verbalize fears and concerns.
- demonstrate effective coping behavior.
- identify a social support network and use available resources.

Nursing Interventions	Rationales
Assess patient and family psychosocial status and adequacy of coping behavior. Document patient and family response.	

Nursing Interventions	Rationales
Provide focused information about condition, plan of care, and environment. Identify a family spokesperson.	Simple and frequent informational updates may reduce fear and anxiety.
Offer reassurance while promoting a realistic perception of condition.	Patients and families in crisis need a sense of hope for optimal recovery.
Provide a simple explanation of VAD function.	The VAD systems are likely to appear overwhelming and complex to a patient and family. Simple explanations of visual and auditory stimuli and possible VAD pumping sensations may reduce anxiety.
Assign consistent nursing and ancillary service caregivers.	Consistency promotes the establishment of an open and trusting relationship between the caregivers and the patient and family.
Conduct frequent multidisciplinary care conferences, including the patient and family when appropriate.	Conferences provide a forum for coordinating a holistic plan of care.
Listen to fears and concerns. Answer questions honestly.	
Encourage unrestricted family visits and family participation in the plan of care.	Unrestricted visiting promotes positive coping.
Implement comfort strategies to reduce pain and anxiety (e.g., pain medication, position changes, skin care, mouth care, control of environmental noise, music).	
Establish an activity/rest schedule. Promote self-care and control over decisions whenever possible. When condition stabilizes, allow undisturbed sleep at night.	Every effort should be made to coordinate care and normalize day and night routines, as this enhances physical and psychological recovery.
Encourage family to personalize the environment with personal possessions, clothing, pictures, and room decorations.	

Nursing Interventions	Rationales
Consult with clinical nurse specialist, chaplain, social worker, financial services, or mental health professional as needed.	
Initiate pretransplant teaching plan when applicable.	Timing and extent of teaching should be determined by clinical status and readiness to learn.
Plan family events when stable (e.g., gatherings, dinners, privacy time, videotaped movies).	
Prepare for transfer from critical care unit when stable: 1. Begin to schedule activities outside of unit (e.g., physical therapy, care conferences, family events, outdoor activities). 2. Provide tour of receiving area. 3. Discuss patient and family fears and concerns related to transfer. 4. Schedule care conference with receiving area. Introduce caregivers.	A stable patient on some types of VAD support may transfer to the intermediate care area while awaiting transplant. Transfer from a familiar staff and a highly monitored critical care unit may be very stressful until relationships are established with new caregivers.
Assist patient and family to prepare for the experience of death when necessary.	In this high-risk patient population, not all patients can be weaned successfully from the VAD or bridged to transplant.

DISCHARGE PLANNING/CONTINUITY OF CARE

- Prepare patient and family for transfer from critical care unit when condition is stable. Discuss concerns and fears.
- Conduct a care conference with the receiving area to coordinate an individualized plan of care. Identify support of key caregivers in transition.
- Assess readiness to learn and initiate a cardiac teaching plan after patient has been successfully weaned from the VAD. Focus on recovery strategies and life-style changes.
- Assess readiness to learn and initiate a cardiac transplant teaching plan. Focus on dealing with the bridge-to-transplant waiting period and life-style changes following transplant.

REFERENCES

English, M. A. (1989). Preventing complications of ventricular assist devices. *Dimensions of Critical Care Nursing, 8*(6), 330–336.

Grady, K. L., Sandiford-Guttenbeil, D. M., & Williams, B. A. (1991). A bridge to transplantation: Mechanical support devices to restore failing circulation. In B. A. Williams, K. L. Grady, & D. M. Sandiford-Guttenbeil (Eds.), *Organ transplantation—A manual for nurses* (pp. 289–317). New York: Springer.

Mulford, E. (1987). Nursing perspectives for the patient receiving postoperative ventricular assistance in the critical care unit. *Heart & Lung, 16,* 246–257.

Quaal, S. J. (Ed.). (1991). Cardiac assist devices. *AACN Clinical Issues in Critical Care Nursing, 2*(3), 475–605.

Teplitz, L. (1990). Patients with ventricular assist devices: Nursing diagnoses. *Dimensions of Critical Care Nursing, 9*(2), 82–87.

Physical and Psychological Rehabilitation

▼

$\mathcal{C}$ARDIAC REHABILITATION

Sandra L. Zemke, RN, BSN

Cardiac Rehabilitation is a three-phase process by which the person with cardiovascular disease is restored to and maintained at the individual's optimal physiological, psychological, social, vocational, and emotional status. Phase I is the hospital inpatient period which lasts from 6 to 14 days for patients with acute myocardial infarction (AMI) or following coronary artery bypass surgery. Rehabilitation is initiated immediately in the form of education and counseling. Exercise in the form of range-of-motion (ROM) activities, intermittent sitting, standing, and walking are performed according to physician referral and at a level determined by the physician or cardiac rehabilitation staff. Phase II cardiac rehabilitation, generally 12 weeks duration, is the convalescent stage beginning within 3 weeks of hospital discharge. This phase takes place in an outpatient cardiac rehabilitation center, usually in a hospital. Emergency equipment and staff who are trained in advanced cardiac life support should be present. Phase III cardiac rehabilitation is an extended, supervised outpatient exercise program, usually in a hospital or clinic setting. This phase is a maintenance phase which may last an extended period of time and does not require telemetry monitoring.

ETIOLOGIES

Cardiac surgery
- Coronary artery bypass grafting
- Heart valve replacement
- Automatic implantable cardioverter defibrillator
- Cardiac transplantation

Coronary artery disease
- AMI
- Cutaneous coronary angioplasty
- Congestive heart failure
- Cardiac dysrhythmia
- Angina

CLINICAL MANIFESTATIONS

The following can occur as a result of poor exercise tolerance:
- elevated pulse rate response to submaximal work
- decreased cardiovascular adaptability to changes in posture
- increased heart rate at rest
- decreased lung volume and vital capacity
- increased incidence of thromboembolism
- muscle atrophy
- fatigue from limited exercise or activity levels
- lightheadedness
- muscular weakness

CLINICAL/DIAGNOSTIC FINDINGS

- Submaximal or maximal exercise testing: Low functional capacity and cardiac ischemia may be present.
- Electrocardiography
  - tachycardia
  - atrial or ventricular ectopy
  - atrial or ventricular enlargement
  - cardiac ischemia
  - myocardial infarction
- Echocardiography
  - atrial, ventricular hypertrophy
  - valvular insufficiency
  - left ventricular wall motion abnormalities
  - decreased left ventricular ejection fraction
- Chest x-Ray
  - congestive changes
  - pleural effusions
  - cardiomegly
- Cardiac catheterization and coronary angiograms
  - decreased cardiac wall motion
  - coronary artery disease detected in the coronary circulation

NURSING DIAGNOSIS: HIGH RISK FOR ACTIVITY INTOLERANCE

Related To acute cardiac event

Risk Factors
- Recent cardiac surgery
- Recent AMI
- Recent cardiac decompensation

Patient Outcomes

Patient will perform exercise and activity at a level of energy expenditure dependent upon tolerance and hemodynamic stability, as evidenced by

- heart rate that does not increase more than 30 beats above the resting heart rate
- telemetry monitoring that displays stable heart rhythm (absence of frequent ventricular dysrhythmias, uncontrolled atrial dysrhythmias, second- or third-degree heart block, symptomatic bradycardia, or tachycardia)
- normal blood pressure response to exercise
- verbalization of feeling well with exercise

Nursing Interventions	Rationales
Review the patient record for the following: 1. past medical history 2. history of present illness 3. social history 4. musculoskeletal or orthopedic limitations 5. pertinent laboratory values [PaO_2, $PaCO_2$, K^+, creatine kinase isoenzyme (CK-MB), hematocrit (Hct)] 6. pertinent tests [chest x-ray, electrocardiogram (ECG), telemetry rhythm]	Prior to treatment the chart is reviewed to determine a plan of care and to determine contraindications to treatment.
Complete cardiac rehabilitation interview with the patient. This includes 1. prior home responsibilities 2. avocational interests 3. exercise habits 4. work history 5. ability to control life's stressors 6. current mental status	The interview allows for an individualized plan of care to be developed.

Nursing Interventions	Rationales

Begin exercises:
1. intensive care unit
  • passive/assistive ROM
  • sitting and standing
  • coughing and deep breathing every hour
2. intermediate care unit
  • upper and lower body calisthenics three times per day
  • graded ambulation with assistance four to six times per day, progress to independent ambulation
  • coughing and deep breathing every hour
	Early exercise following an acute cardiac event is used as a means for preventing complications of bedrest and the deconditioning that accompanies it.

Monitor heart rate and blood pressure and observe telemetry for hemodynamic stability with progressive exercise.	These measures reflect that progressive exercise is being well tolerated.

NURSING DIAGNOSIS: KNOWLEDGE DEFICIT

Related To new medical/surgical condition and lack of previous exposure to cardiac problem

Defining Characteristics
Verbalization indicating inadequate understanding of desired health behaviors
Inability to identify and modify behaviors

Patient Outcomes
Patient will
• verbalize home exercise and activity guidelines.
• identify personal cardiac risk factors.
• have a plan for modifying cardiac risk factors.

Nursing Interventions	**Rationales**
Assess readiness to learn and teach appropriate content regarding 1. anatomy and physiology of current cardiac diagnosis 2. controllable cardiac risk factors (smoking, hypertension, hyperlipidemia, lack of aerobic exercise, obesity, stress, diabetes) 3. strategies for life-style modification for applicable risk factors.	Knowledge enables the patient to make heart healthy choices in the future, continuing the benefits of cardiac rehabilitation.
Collaborate with appropriate staff to assist in developing strategies for change: 1. Dietician will instruct in a low-fat, low-cholesterol diet or other restrictions as needed. 2. Physical therapy and occupational therapy will assist with increasing exercise and activity levels.	
Discuss exercise program prior to discharge. This includes: 1. frequency 2. intensity 3. duration 4. appropriate modes of exercise 5. review pulse counting and exercise target heart rate 6. signs and symptoms of exercise intolerance 7. rationale for a life time cardiovascular exercise program	During discussion individual problems can be addressed.
Review individualized activity home program prior to discharge. This includes: 1. current restrictions 2. guidelines for progressing activity to normal levels	Patients will be more confident regarding activities if they understand specific recommendations.

DISCHARGE PLANNING/CONTINUITY OF CARE

Refer to a phase II cardiac rehabilitation program to continue with supervised exercise and life-style modification. The patient will receive the following:

- individualized exercise prescription
- telemetry monitoring to detect arrhythmias during progressive exercise
- a typical exercise session which includes 10 min of warm-up calisthenics and stretching, 30 min of aerobic exercise, usually using the treadmill and stationary bike, and 5 min of cool-down calisthenics and stretching
- cardiac risk factor education and counseling in the form of group education as well as one-to-one counseling to promote behavior change

During this phase of rehabilitation the patient can begin practicing appropriate behavior changes which will promote heart health.

REFERENCES

American Association of Cardiovascular and Pulmonary Rehabilitation. (1991). *Guidelines for cardiac rehabilitation programs.* Champaign, IL: Human Kinetics Publishers.

Fardy, P. S., Yanowitz, F. G., & Wilson, P. K. (1988). *Cardiac rehabilitation, adult fitness, and exercise testing.* Philadelphia: Lea & Febiger.

Pashkow, F., Pashkow, P., Schafer, M., & Ferguson, C. (1988). *Successful cardiac rehabilitation.* Loveland, CO: Heartwatchers.

*C*OPING WITH CARDIAC CRISES

Rita E. Herman, RN, MSN

A crisis is a state of disequilibrium which results from an imbalance between a patient's perception of a stressful event or situation and the patient's current coping strategies and external supports and resources to deal with the stressful event/situation. The heart is thought of as the essence of physical and emotional well-being as well as a symbol for love and life. Thus, psychological crises are quite common with any cardiac problem.

ETIOLOGIES

- Environmental stressors produced by hospital structure
  - coercion
  - personal space invasions
  - regimented routine
  - lack of control, power, authority, attention
  - loss of dignity
  - lack of individuation
  - cultural differences
- Inadequate personal resources
  - physical
  - mental/emotional
  - cognitive
  - sensory
  - perceptual
  - spiritual
- Lack of supportive social network
- Memories of past stressful experiences or events
- Perceived or actual threats
  - to: safety, security, self-concept, values, beliefs, goal attainment
  - of: disease process, life-style of helplessness, terminal illness, death
  - to change in: role, socioeconomic status, health status
- Continued stress over time

CLINICAL MANIFESTATIONS

- Depression
- Inappropriate aggression
- Manipulation

- Anxiety
- Powerlessness
- Noncompliance

NURSING DIAGNOSIS: HIGH RISK FOR INEFFECTIVE INDIVIDUAL COPING AND DEPRESSION

Risk Factors
- Life-threatening disease process
- Belief that illness or stress are uncontrollable
- Lack or inadequacy of internal coping strategies and/or external resources and supports

Patient Outcomes
Patient will demonstrate effective coping behaviors, as evidenced by
- adequate problem solving and decision making
- appropriate interpersonal interactions with staff and significant others
- higher energy level and motivation for activities of daily living and participation in the recovery process
- participation in defining goals, activities, and outcomes
- congruence of affect with event
- absence of suicidal thoughts and feelings
- congruence with physical complaints and current physical status
- diminished sleeplessness and appetite disturbance
- appropriate orientation
- lack of confusion
- congruence with level of independence and physical status

Nursing Interventions	Rationales
Assess suicide potential in hospital setting by evaluating health history, family history, support systems, presence of vegetative symptoms, presence of thought disorders and previous thoughts, feelings, and/or attempts:	Suicide is the most serious complication of depression as it is truly life threatening.
1. Assess impact of current stressor by evaluating current plan for self-harm.	

Nursing Interventions	Rationales
2. Identify strategies patient will use when suicidal thoughts and/or feelings occur.	
3. Contract with patient to not harm self.	
4. If patient is unable to contract, arrange for a sitter.	
5. Assess and observe for physical systems.	Physical symptoms can contribute to intensity and chronicity of depression.
Assess sleep patterns: 1. Assess reasons for sleeplessness 2. Teach relaxation techniques 3. Offer sedation if not contraindicated 4. Decrease number of interruptions during night and assist with establishing appropriate sleep-wake cycle.	Patient who is exhausted from lack of sleep has depleted energy to participate in the physical recovery activities, and thus depression may remain or become exacerbated.
Assess eating patterns: 1. Encourage and supervise proper nutrition 2. Determine favorite foods and ask family or significant others to participate as resources for these.	Patient who is undernourished has depleted energy to participate in the physical recovery activities, and thus depression may remain or become exacerbated.
Assess the meaning of the patient's perception of the current stressful, cardiac event. Examples of appropriate questions are: "What does this current situation mean to you?" "What do you think is going to happen?" "What would you like to see happen?" "What else is going on in your life currently?" "Tell me about some other crises in your life and how you handled these."	It is the patient's perception of the event that matters. If there have been or are other stresses, they may also contribute to the degree of depression. This assists with understanding what the patient is experiencing.

Nursing Interventions	Rationales
Assess the patient's current perception of reality for distortions. If distortions are present, supply accurate information and pose alternatives. Discuss alternate interpretations of the present events and determine if there is a meaning or rationale for the distortion.	Once the nurse understands the distortion, the patient can be helped with understanding the inaccuracy of the perception and link to depression.
Encourage patient to participate in self-care regimen congruent with physical status: 1. Structure schedule with patient's participation. 2. Give positive reinforcement.	Exercise, social contacts outside of confines of hospital room, and participation in activities of daily living enhance self-worth and independence.
Help the patient see the relationship between the depressive symptoms and the current situation.	Patients are often relieved to see the connection between the current situation and symptoms they are experiencing.
Assist the patient to recognize, understand, and ventilate feelings:	Verbalization of feelings helps establish a therapeutic relationship.
1. Use an empathetic approach to help the patient identify feelings.	The patient can verbalize thoughts and feelings and connect them to the current situation.
2. Observe and give feedback on the verbal and nonverbal expression of feelings: for example, "You look angry, are you?" "It sounds like you feel hopeless right now." "How do you feel about what has happened to you?"	Acceptance shown by the nurse enhances self-acceptance in the patient.
3. Connect the feeling to the content: for example, "You feel hopeless because so much has happened to you in a short period of time and you feel like you are going backward instead of forward."	This connection helps the patient develop a more realistic perception of self and events.

Nursing Interventions	Rationales
4. Tell the patient how others have felt in similar situations.	This helps the patient understand universality and realization that "I'm not alone." "I'm not the only person who has felt like this."
Assist the patient to identify and utilize supportive resources: "Who are the supportive people in your life?" "Who has helped you in the past?" "Who could be helpful to you now?"	The more the patient is involved in this process, the more likely he or she will take the action required.
Administer antidepressants as prescribed.	Antidepressants can assist the patient with establishing adequate sleep and appetite to attain an energy level and motivation to actively work on problems and issues.
Involve the patient in discharge planning: 1. Talk with the patient about things he or she is looking forward to doing once home and people he or she enjoys being with. 2. Encourage the patient to talk about potential problems and discuss coping strategies.	The more the patient is involved in the process, the more he or she will feel that discharge will be a reality and that there is "life after hospitalization."

NURSING DIAGNOSIS: HIGH RISK FOR ANXIETY

Risk Factors
- Unexpected hospitalization
- Length of hospitalization
    - too short due to insurance restrictions
    - too long compared to average length of stay for a specific cardiac event
- Delayed goal achievement in the cardiac rehabilitation process
- Lack of or inadequacy of coping strategies
- Fear of outcome

Patient Outcomes
Patient will demonstrate, both verbally and behaviorally, a decrease in anxiety, as evidenced by

- accurate sensory perception
- alertness and ability to concentrate
- self-insight and observation
- accurate observation of events in environment
- ability to make connections between events and verbalize them
- ability to learn

Nursing Interventions	Rationales
During mild or moderate anxiety: Help patient name the feeling. Have patient describe the events that occurred that may be related to the anxiety. Help the patient connect the anxiety to unmet expectations. Help the patient determine what he or she needs to reduce or relieve the anxiety through the problem-solving process.	The process of talking with a nurse and feeling understood by another person often helps alleviate or reduce anxiety. Additionally, self-understanding and connecting the anxiety and events that triggered it, assist with bringing relief. Patients may need more information, a talk with the physician, additional sleep, or just reassurance.
Assist the patient with getting what he or she needs from self and others to relieve or reduce the anxiety: 1. Teach assertive communication skills. 2. Teach progressive muscle relaxation and imagery.	
During severe or extreme anxiety: Remain with patient. Speak in calm manner. Provide reassurance for safety and security. Offer sedation if needed.	This level of anxiety is quite frightening to the patient and usually the patient responds well to talking with someone and having someone stay with them to enhance safety and security and provide reassurance. When anxiety level decreases, then utilize nursing interventions for mild or moderate anxiety.

NURSING DIAGNOSIS: HIGH RISK FOR VIOLENCE

Risk Factors
- Frustration
- Fear

- Loss of dignity
- Perceived threat
- Thwarting of goals
- Thwarting of needs for power, control, authority, attention

Patient Outcomes

Patient will be free of aggression, as evidenced by
- appropriate goal-directed, problem-solving behavior
- utilization of assertive communication
- demonstrating respect for personal integrity of others

Nursing Interventions	Rationales
Assist patient with identification and expression of feelings and/or threats by developing a relationship with patient in which he or she can verbalize anger, frustration, and fear:	Identification of feelings is the first step in helping the patient channel them appropriately.
1. Provide feedback on nonverbal behavior to assist with underlying anger, frustration, or fear.	
2. Help patient identify sources of anger, frustration, or fear.	Identifying sources assists patients with realizing they have a choice about how they feel.
3. Assist the patient with identifying acceptable methods of expressing anger.	All feelings are acceptable but all behavior is not.
4. Point out consequences for self and others of inappropriate aggressions.	
5. Help patient with anxiety reduction.	Anxiety reduction will decrease the potential for inappropriate aggressive behavior.

Nursing Interventions	Rationales
Prevent injury to self and others and recognize potential for inappropriate aggression: 1. Tell patient you want to help him or her regain and maintain control.	An interactive, positive one-to-one relationship with a patient will be helpful in preventing inappropriate aggressive behavior.
2. Attempt to "talk down" by helping patient verbalize what he or she is experiencing along with feelings.	
3. Set limits gently.	
4. Be aware of and identify potentially stressful situations for that particular patient and be available to patient during those periods.	
5. Respect patient's need for personal space.	
6. Provide explanation of events that will affect patient and be truthful.	
7. Avoid arguments and allow patient to assist with maintaining some control over daily schedule by including him or her in the decision-making process.	
8. Determine need for medications and physical restraints.	Ongoing assessment of appropriate outcomes of verbal and nonverbal interactions is important so that medications and/or physical restraints can be utilized to prevent injury to patient and staff.

NURSING DIAGNOSIS: HIGH RISK FOR POWERLESSNESS

Risk Factors
- Threat to physical integrity
- Hospitalization
- Loss of control

Patient Outcomes

Patient will be able to control some activities and outcomes in current situations, as exhibited by
- verbalization of feelings of having some control
- demonstration of adequate coping skills by expressing feelings and being involved in appropriate decision-making and self-care

Nursing Interventions	Rationales
Individualize daily routine. Be attentive to patient's communication. Provide for basic needs with encouragement of choice and increase in self-care as patient progress warrants. Maintain patient's interest in treatment and recovery.	As patients realize they can control or at least influence certain outcomes by active decision making and participation, powerlessness seems to diminish. Patients feel less overwhelmed and dependent in that process.
Show willingness to be adaptable and flexible to increase patient's independence, power, and control.	
Assist patient in identifying feelings of powerlessness.	
Help patient differentiate between situations that can be changed and those that cannot.	
Help patient set realistic goals for self.	
Identify aspects of hospitalization and self-care that patient can control and structure opportunities for patient to participate and succeed. Encourage questions about self-care and teach.	

NURSING DIAGNOSIS: HIGH RISK FOR DEFENSIVE COPING

Risk Factors
- Anxiety
- Compromised physical status
- Dependence on others to meet needs
- Powerlessness and lack of control in certain situations

Patient Outcomes

Patient will be free of manipulative behavior, as evidenced by
- discussion of factors and issues which promote manipulative behavior
- relating to caregivers in an assertive manner to effectively communicate feelings, needs, and desires

Nursing Interventions	Rationales
Assist patient with defining rights and responsibilities within the hospital setting. Assist patient with examination of manipulative behaviors in a nonjudgmental manner as well as providing constructive feedback.	Patients change their view of themselves and no longer think of themselves as victims when rights and responsibilities are defined and they know how to effectively communicate to get their needs met.
Assist patients with assertive communication skills to communicate feelings, thoughts, needs, and wants.	
Formulate a care plan with patient participation and discuss appropriate response time to needs and wants.	Patients will have a clear understanding of the guidelines and expectations as well as definition of activities he or she can accomplish independently. Also, health care team members can be consistent in their response to patients.

NURSING DIAGNOSIS: HIGH RISK FOR INEFFECTIVE MANAGEMENT OF THERAPEUTIC REGIMEN

Risk Factors
- Lack of understanding or information about disease, physical status, and treatment regimen
- Poor relationship with health care team members
- Lack of financial or supportive resources
- No obvious improvement with current treatment regimen
- History of negative experiences with health care system
- Denial of current health status.

Patient Outcomes

Patient will effectively manage the therapeutic regimen, as evidenced by
- verbalization of understanding of treatment regimen
- maintenance of ongoing dialogue with health care team members

- keeping appointments with health care team professionals
- taking scheduled medications
- absence of signs and symptoms or complications related to disease process that are within patient's control

Nursing Interventions	Rationales
Assess patient's willingness and intent to follow ongoing treatment activities by behavior in hospital setting.	
Assess adequacy of financial supportive and pragmatic resources (e.g., transportation to physician's office) and assist with defining alternate resources if necessary.	Having comprehensive information about patients and significant others allows caregivers to assist with a plan to enhance compliance with treatment.
Assist patient with knowledge base and understanding of treatment regime related to illness and physical status.	Information enhances understanding and contributes to compliance.
Explore patients' and significant others' attitudes, belief system, and understanding of patient's current status and appropriate treatment.	Meeting patients and significant others at their level and progressing from there contributes to a situation where everyone is at the same place at the same time.
Establish a trusting relationship with patient.	Being honest and direct about a patient's illness and expectations related to the treatment regime on an onging basis is important in establishing trust.
Discuss fears and concerns about illness and treatment regime.	
Clearly specify and document treatment plan and instructions and patients' responsibilities.	If patients are included in the process and their understanding is accurate related to the outcome of compliance versus noncompliance, problem solving to enhance compliance will be more readily utilized.
Provide patient with specific guidelines to monitor progress.	
Discuss consequences of noncompliance.	

Nursing Interventions	Rationales
If ineffective behaviors persist, discuss possible reasons and underlying issues with patient and significant others.	

DISCHARGE PLANNING/CONTINUITY OF CARE

- Teach patients what to expect from the health care system.
- Teach patients what is expected of them.
- Educate patients about their illness, treatment, and prognosis.
- Assist patients to develop problem-solving techniques and coping skills.
- Alert patients to the signs, symptoms, and situations when they need to call the health care team for assistance or intervention.
- Inform patient of support groups in the community.

REFERENCES

Aguilera, D. C., & Messick, J. (1990). *Crisis intervention: Theory and methodology.* St. Louis, MO: Mosby.

American Psychiatric Association. (1987). *Diagnostic and statistical manual of mental disorders,* (3rd rev. ed.). Washington, DC.

Badger, T. A. (1990). Men with cardiovascular disease and their spouses: Coping, health and marital adjustment. *Archives of Psychiatric Nursing,* 4(5), 319–324.

Beck, A. T. (1972). *Depression, causes and treatment.* Philadelphia: University of Pennsylvania Press.

Carson, R. C., & Butcher, J. N. (1992). *Abnormal psychology and modern life* (9th ed.). New York: HarperCollins.

Haber, J., Leach, A. M., Schudy, S. M., & Sideleau, B. F. (1992). *Comprehensive psychiatric nursing* (4th ed.). New York: McGraw-Hill.

Turnbull, J., Aitkin, L., Black, L., & Patterson, B. (1991). Turn it around: Short-term management for aggression and anger. *Journal of Psychosocial Nursing,* 28(6), 6–10.

Whitley, G. G. (1991). Ritualistic behaviors: Breaking the cycle. *Journal of Psychosocial Nursing,* 29(10), 31–35.

INDEX

Note: Page numbers followed by t indicate tables

A

Accelerated junction rhythm, following cardiac surgery, 201t
Activase, in thrombolytic therapy, 34–37
Activity intolerance, and infective endocarditis, 123–124
Acute myocardial infarction, 11–29
  acute pain and, 12–16
  altered tissue perfusion and, 24–25
  anxiety and, 25–28
  clinical findings, 11–12
  clinical manifestations, 11
  decreased cardiac output and, 16–23
  diagnostic findings, 11–12
  etiologies, 11
  knowledge deficit and, 28–29
  thrombolytic therapy and, 30–49.
    See also Thrombolytic therapy
Adjustment, impaired, and implantable cardioverter defibrillator, 262–263
Adrenalin, in cardiogenic shock, 98t
Aggression, patient, 298–300
Airway clearance, ineffective, and aortic aneurysm repair, 231–232
Alteplase, 34–37
Amiloride, in congestive heart failure, 79t
Amines, sympathomimetic, in cardiogenic shock, 98t
Amoxicillin, in infective endocarditis, 127t
Amrinone
  in cardiomyopathy and myocarditis, 106
  in congestive heart failure, 81t
Analgesic medications, in acute myocardial infarction, 13, 16

Aneurysm repair, aortic. *See* Aortic aneurysm repair
Angina pectoris, 3–10
  acute pain and, 9–10
  altered tissue perfusion and, 5, 8
  antianginal drugs and, 6t–7t
  clinical findings, 4
  clinical manifestations, 3–4
  continuity of care, 10
  decreased cardiac output and, 4–5
  diagnostic findings, 4
  discharge planning and, 10
  etiologies, 3
  impaired gas exchange and, 8–9
  percutaneous transluminal coronary angioplasty and, 52
Angioplasty. *See* Percutaneous transluminal coronary angioplasty
Angiotensin converting enzyme inhibitors
  in cardiomyopathy and myocarditis, 106
  in congestive heart failure, 80t
Anorexia. *See* Nutrition, altered
Antianginal medications, in acute myocardial infarction, 13
Antibiotic medications, in infective endocarditis, 119, 127t
Anticoagulant medications
  in acute myocardial infarction, 25
  in cardiomyopathy and myocarditis, 106
  in cerebral vascular accident, 143t
Antidepressant medications, in psychological crises, 297
Antidysrhythmic medications, 23t